The Inescapable Immune Escape Pandemic

Nobody Can Conceal The Science
That Nature Is Now Desperate To Unveil

Society In Highly Vaccinated Countries
Will Be Caught By Surprise

Geert Vanden Bossche, DVM, PHD

The Inescapable Immune
Escape Pandemic

Nobody Can Conceal The Science
That Nature Is Now Desperate To Unveil

Society In Highly Vaccinated Countries
Will Be Caught By Surprise

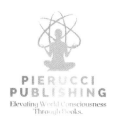

PIERUCCI
PUBLISHING
Elevating World Consciousness
Through Books.

Pierucci Publishing books may be purchased in bulk at special discounts for sales promotion, corporate gifts, fund-raising, or educational purposes. Special editions can be created to specifications. For details, contact the Special Sales Department, Pierucci Publishing, PO Box 8067, Aspen, CO 81612.

Publishing@PierucciPublishing.com

Visit our website at www.pieruccipublishing.com.

Paperback ISBN: 978-1-956257-69-4
Ebook ISBN: 978-1-956257-79-3
Hardcover ISBN: 978-1-956257-80-9

Cover Design by Stephanie Pierucci
Edited by Bart Provost & John Heathco
Geert's portrait by Berten.be

Library of Congress Control Number: 2023931753

Dedication

Dedicated to all those who could not hear, read or
understand my predictions.

Acknowledgements

To my friend John Heathco, whose relentless support has been invaluable in completing this book. In the two years that we have collaborated together, John has evolved from a computer engineer to somebody who holds a deep understanding of the evolutionary dynamics of the pandemic. He's a textbook example of intellectual diligence in a world of crippling intellectual laziness. His comprehension of immunology, vaccinology, virology and evolutionary biology comes on the back of being a curious mind. In fact, his intelligent questions have helped me improve my own insights and understanding of the pandemic dynamics. I am indebted to John for editing, correcting, fine-tuning and even addressing flaws in my scientific phrasing for this manuscript. John, I couldn't have written this book without you. You're my hero.

To my friend Dr. Rob Rennebohm. Dr. Rennebohm is an exceptional person who combines excelling knowledge in the medical field with wholehearted intentions. Not only is he knowledgeable about immunology and childhood diseases, but he possesses a unique skill in writing about complex problems in a way that is accessible to the wide audience of lay readers. His 'Open Letter to Parents and Pediatricians Regarding COVID Vaccination' (on my website at https://www.voiceforscienceandsolidarity.org/ is just one example of his ability to pair deep professional insights with exceptional writing skills.

To my friend Bart Provost. Bart has been reliable, fast and efficient with technical and logistic support, including managing the contracts and operations that made this book possible. Bart is a pillar in my organization Voice For Science and Solidarity https://www.voiceforscienceandsolidarity.org/, and ensures that our many initiatives, including this book, are executed to completion.
To Stephanie Pierucci, who was kind enough to help materialize this initiative as soon as she heard about it. Her support with editing, publishing and ensuring wide dissemination of this book is highly

appreciated. Putting the public (health) interest above financial interest has become rare these days, but Stephanie has shown commitment to that.

To my family. Thank you to Johanna and my children for having been a harbor of peace, rest and love during these difficult times, which included harassment, vilification, gaslighting and berating. I thank them for their patience, unwavering confidence, respect, and trust in me. Their continuous support and appreciation made me strong enough to withstand every storm I've weathered.

To my followers. Thank you for your encouraging words, friendship, trust, and for making valuable resources available.

Last, but not least, I thank all those who continue to consider me sane, despite my very unusual predictions.

Publisher's Note

you. This book provides content related to physical and/or health issues. As such, use of this book implies your acceptance of this disclaimer.

What people are saying about 'The Inescapable Immune Escape Pandemic' by Geert Vanden Bossche

The complexity of the human immune system is something to be admired - and Geert Vanden Bossche certainly does. He has the soul of a true scientist: an investigator - exploring all possibilities (however unlikely! to seek answers and truths concerning the potential devastating effects of mass injection campaigns using novel products during a pandemic. As he states in Chapter 11, and I agree, it was never a question of *if* variants of concern would emerge, but *when*. Geert's book is a call to action and a guidebook - the COVID-19 injection campaign must be brought to a complete halt, and investigations done to prevent this from happening again. And as Geert summarizes so aptly in Chapter 9: "Nature mercilessly punishes man's incredibly naive belief that through technology, he can control biology." I completely agree.

Dr. Jessica Rose
PHD, MSc., BSc.

The first to inform the WHO of the folly of mass vaccination against C19, the first to explain why failure was inevitable, why death and sickness would rise not fall as a result, Dr Vanden Bossche now lays out his stall for all to see and decipher. This unique book reads as much like an adventure novel as it does a scientific treatise, one that's both erudite and accessible. Most of all, it blows a gaping hole through the rationale used to justify the largest, uncontrolled human experiment ever conducted. It's essential reading for anyone who cares about humanity.

Robert Verkerk PHD
Founder, Executive & Scientific Director, Alliance for Natural Health International

Geert Vanden Bossche's book on the SARS-CoV-2 pandemic is a must-read for anyone looking to understand the potential consequences of human intervention with vaccines based upon novel technology. His previous predictions for the pandemic have proven to be incredibly accurate, and his deep & comprehensive analysis on how immune escape will further unfold is both enlightening and sobering. This is a book that will challenge your assumptions and leave you better prepared for the future.

John Heathco
Computer Engineer & Serial Entrepreneur

List of Abbreviations

(h)ACE2	(human) Angiotensin-Converting Enzyme 2
Ab	Antibody
ACE2	angiotensin-converting enzyme 2
Ag	Antigen
AIESD	Antibody-Independent Enhancement of Severe Covid-19 Disease
APC	Antigen-Presenting Cell
BCR	B-Cell Receptor
C-19	Covid-19
CBII	Cell-Based Innate Immunity
CBIIS	Cell-Based Innate Immune System
CoV	Coronavirus
CTL	Cytotoxic T-Lymphocyte

DC	Dendritic Cell
DMS	Deep Mutational Scanning
EOSV(s)	Early Omicron-derived SubVariant(s)
LRT	Lower Respiratory Tract
NBTI	Natural Breakthrough Infection
NK cell	Natural killer cell
OOV	Original Omicron Variant
pNAb(s)	potentially Neutralizing Antibody (Antibodies)
PNNAb(s)	Polyreactive Non-Neutralizing Antibody (Antibodies)
S-RBD	Receptor-Binding Domain of Spike protein
S-NTD	N-terminal domain within Spike protein
SC-2	SARS-CoV-2
SIR	Steric Immune Refocusing
TCR	T-Cell Receptor

URT	Upper Respiratory Tract
VBTI	Vaccine Breakthrough Infection

Glossary of Terms

Breakthrough Infection (BTI)

> For the purpose of this manuscript, SC-2 **breakthrough infection** (BTI) relates to enhanced productive SC-2 infection and Covid-19 (C-19) disease in previously productively infected- or C-19-vaccinated individuals.

Cell-Based Innate Immune system (CBIIS):

> For the purpose of this manuscript, the **cell-based innate immune system** refers to the cellular components of the innate immune system that specifically recognize pathogen-infected or otherwise pathologically altered host cells and have the capacity to eliminate those cells. The principal cell type of the CBIIS *sensu stricto* is the Natural Killer cell (NK cell).

Cytolytic Killing of Virus-Infected Cells

> For the purpose of this manuscript, **cytolytic killing of virus-infected cells** is defined as cytolysis of SC-2-infected target host cells by MHC (Major Histocompatibility Complex) class I -unrestricted cytotoxic lymphocytes (CTLs) as a result of enhanced uptake of pNAb-complexed progeny virions into tissue-resident APCs.

Early Omicron-derived Subvariants (EOSVs)

> For the purpose of this manuscript, **early Omicron-derived subvariants** refer to Omicron BA.2 and its early descendants, e.g., BA.4/5, BA.2.12.1, BA.2.11 and BA.2.9.1.

Highly (or largely) C-19 vaccinated or high C-19 vaccine coverage rate

> For the purpose of this manuscript, **highly (or largely) C-19 vaccinated or high C-19 vaccine coverage rate** refers to a high rate of C-19 vaccinations with mRNA-based vaccines (regardless of the number of injections/doses or combination with other, non-mRNA-based C-19 vaccines)

or to a high rate of C-19 priming with non-mRNA vaccines followed by one or more booster injections.

Infection-Inhibiting Abs

For the purpose of this manuscript, **infection-inhibiting Abs** refers to non-hACE2-competing Abs that are capable of preventing viral infection.

Non-Productive Infections

For the purpose of this manuscript, **non-productive infections** are SC-2 infections that are controlled/contained at an early stage of the infection (i.e., before viral progeny is produced) due to strong cell-based innate immunity (CBII). Non-productive infections are asymptomatic.

PNNAb-dependent breakthrough infection

For the purpose of this manuscript, **PNNAb-dependent breakthrough infection (*PNNAb-dependent BTI*)** is defined as breakthrough SC-2 infection that is triggered by polyreactive non-neutralizing Abs (PNNAbs).

PNNAb-dependent natural breakthrough infection

For the purpose of this manuscript, **PNNAb-dependent natural breakthrough infection (*PNNAb-dependent NBTI*)** is defined as PNNAb-dependent BTI in previously infection-primed individuals.

PNNAb-dependent vaccine breakthrough infection

For the purpose of this manuscript, **PNNAb-dependent vaccine breakthrough infection (*PNNAb-dependent VBTI*)** is defined as PNNAb-dependent BTI in previously vaccine-primed individuals.

PNNAb- or Ab-independent vaccine breakthrough infection

For the purpose of this manuscript, **PNNAb- or Ab-independent vaccine breakthrough infection ([PNN]Ab-independent VBTI)** is defined as VBTI that is not triggered by PNNAbs or other Abs but instead mediated by a high level of intrinsic viral infectiousness.

Productive infection

For the purpose of this manuscript, **productive infection** refers to a SC-2 infection that leads to at least one reproductive cycle of the virus

Sidelining of the cell-based innate immune system (CBIIS)

For the purpose of this manuscript, **sidelining of the CBIIS** relates to failure of the CBIIS to eliminate SC-2 virus-infected host cells at an early stage of infection due to enhanced (PNNAb-dependent or -independent) viral infectiousness. Repeated exposure to SC-2 immune escape variants in the presence of vaccinal Abs makes sidelining of the CBIIS (during a pandemic of immune escape variants) irreversible.

Steric Immune Refocusing (SIR)

For the purpose of this manuscript, **steric immune refocusing (SIR)** is defined as re-orientation of the humoral S-directed immune response towards more conserved, immune subdominant S-associated epitopes as a result of steric masking of variable, immunodominant S protein-associated epitopes by pre-existing, low-affinity pNAbs.

Vaccinee

For the purpose of this manuscript, **vaccinee** refers to an individual who has received one or more C-19 vaccine injections.

Viral Immune Escape Pandemic

For the purpose of this manuscript, a **viral immune escape pandemic** refers to a viral pandemic that is characterized by a (rapid) succession of dominantly circulating or co-circulating viral immune escape variants.

Viral Infectivity

For the purpose of this manuscript, **viral infectivity** relates to the capacity of a virus to cause infection in a susceptible population.

Viral Infectiousness

For the purpose of this manuscript, **viral infectiousness** relates to the capacity of a viral particle to enter a susceptible host cell and exploit its resources to replicate and produce progeny infectious viral particles, which may lead to infection.

(Virus-) Neutralizing Antibodies (NAbs)

For the purpose of this manuscript, **(virus-) neutralizing antibodies** relate to antibodies (Abs) that are capable of inhibiting viral infection by preventing epitopes comprised within S-RBD (the receptor-binding domain of SARS-CoV-2 spike protein) from binding to human ACE2 (*angiotensin-converting enzyme 2*).

Trans infection

***Trans* infection** relates to a productive infection of target cells by SC-2 virions that are carried on the surface of DCs and which is triggered by binding of S surface-expressed N-linked glycans to C-type lectin receptors expressed on the surface of DCs in a way that promotes exposure of a polypeptide domain within NTD that is capable of binding to sialogangliosides comprised within lipid rafts of target cell membranes. This interaction would enable fusogenic rearrangement of spike protein and hence, facilitate attachment of the receptor-binding motif to the ACE2 receptor.

Trans fusion

Trans fusion relates to ACE2-independent cell-to-cell fusion between a SC-2-infected and a non-infected neighboring cell, thereby resulting in the formation of syncytia and promoting cell-to-cell spread of infection in the target organ

Preliminary Comments

As trained CBII has broadly virus-sterilizing capacity and is an intrinsic component of naturally induced immunity, immunity induced by SC-2 infection in healthy individuals[1] is always more effective than vaccine-induced humoral immunity in preventing or controlling productive infection and transmission upon subsequent exposure to viral variants.

As trained innate immunity is SC-2 variant-nonspecific and can rapidly adapt and react via epigenetic imprinting to changes in the host environment, a trained CBIIS largely protects against productive infection upon subsequent exposure to more infectious SC-2 variants. This is in sharp contrast to infection- or vaccine-elicited spike protein (S-specific Abs. As exposure to heterologous SC-2 variants in the presence of elevated titers of sub functional Abs promotes immune escape, it is not surprising that S-specific Ab titers induced by natural productive infection rapidly decline (as the CBIIS normally eliminates a substantial part of the viral load at an early stage of infection. This also allows for a swift recall of memory B cells that produce high Ab titers upon re-exposure while avoiding steric immune refocusing (chapter 1.2.3.

For the purpose of this manuscript, SC-2 'productive infections' are SC-2 infections that lead to at least one reproductive cycle of the virus. Productive infections can either be rapidly controlled by the CBIIS and therefore be *mild,* or they cannot be controlled by the CBIIS and lead to more extensive replication with multiple replication cycles before being controlled by the adaptive immune system. Productive SC-2 infections that break through the CBIIS but are rapidly (i.e., after about one week controlled by the adaptive immune system typically cause *moderate* Covid-19 (C-19 disease. However, C-19 disease that cannot be rapidly controlled by the adaptive immune system is likely to progress to *severe* C-19 disease.

For the purpose of this manuscript, SC-2 'breakthrough infection' (BTI relates to enhanced productive SC-2 infection and C-19 disease in previously productively infected- or C-19-vaccinated individuals.

As BTIs imply the presence of pre-existing Abs that bind with low affinity to the circulating SC-variant, classical Ab-dependent enhancement of disease (ADE) does not qualify as BTI[2]. ADE requires the virus to hijack Fc receptor-bearing myeloid cells such as monocytes, macrophages, dendritic cells and use them as target cells for viral replication instead of APCs (ref. 1).

For the purpose of this manuscript, '*PNNAb-dependent BTIs*' are defined as breakthrough SC-2 infections that are triggered by polyreactive non-neutralizing Abs (PNNAbs). PNNAb-dependent BTIs occur in the presence of pre-existing *neutralizing Abs* (NAbs) that have strongly diminished neutralizing capacity towards a more infectious, antigenically shifted SC-2 variant (hence, called '*potentially neutralizing Abs*'; pNAbs). By binding to the antigenic S variant expressed on the surface of heterologous SC-2 virus, pNAbs are thought to trigger changes in colloidal viral properties that lead to the formation of weak viral aggregates and thereby stimulate the production of PNNAbs. PNNAbs have been reported to facilitate BTI by rendering vaccinated individuals more susceptible to productive SC-2 infection. Enhanced susceptibility to productive infection is thought to be due to enhanced ACE2 (Angiotensin-converting enzyme 2)-mediated entry of viral particles into susceptible host cells (so-called '*PNNAb-dependent enhancement of viral infectiousness*') [refs. 2, 3 and 4].

PNNAb-dependent BTIs may occur upon exposure of previously infection- or C-19 vaccine-primed individuals to poorly neutralizable, antigenically shifted SC-2 immune escape variants. For the purpose of this manuscript, PNNAb-dependent BTIs in previously infection-primed individuals are referred to as 'PNNAb-dependent natural BTIs' (*PNNAb-dependent NBTIs*) whereas PNNAb-dependent BTIs in previously vaccine-primed individuals are referred to as '*PNNAb-dependent vaccine BTIs*' (*PNNAb-dependent VBTIs*). As PNNAbs suppress viral virulence, PNNAb-dependent BTIs do not cause severe C-19 disease. However, not all BTIs that are associated with protection against severe C-19 disease are mediated by PNNAbs. For example, SC-2 variants with high intrinsic infectiousness may cause BTIs that are not triggered by

PNNAbs or other Abs. For the purpose of this manuscript, such BTIs are referred to as '*PNNAb- or Ab-independent VBTIs*'.

For the purpose of this manuscript, '*steric immune refocusing (SIR)*' is defined as re-orientation of the humoral S-directed immune response towards more conserved, immune subdominant S-associated epitopes as a result of steric masking of variable, immunodominant S protein-associated epitopes by pre-existing, low-affinity pNAbs. This mechanism occurs when pre-existing vaccine-induced anti-S pNAbs bind with low affinity to S protein. Instead of recalling previously imprinted anti-S immune responses, S-associated immunodominant epitopes will bind to these pre-existing, low-affinity pNAbs. Binding of the latter masks the S-associated immunodominant epitopes and thereby causes steric hindrance to their immune recognition. This allows the immune system to skew the immune response towards new, immune subdominant epitopes (fig. 3.

Because the re-directed Abs have relatively low affinity, their neutralizing capacity is relatively low. However, it seems likely that previously vaccine-primed noncognate T helper cells foster continuing maturation of *de novo* primed memory B cells in germinal centers (refs. 29, 30 and 31. Enhanced maturation of these cells would eventually result in production of broadly neutralizing Abs that are characterized by a much higher level of affinity. However, it has been reported that further maturation of these noncognate Th-dependent memory B cells can take several months (refs. 29, 30 and 31. In the meantime, short-lived broadly cross-neutralizing Abs of low affinity exert enhanced immune pressure on the targeted subdominant cross-neutralizing epitopes and thereby drive immune escape (chapters 1.2.1.-1.2.4.

For the purpose of this manuscript, '*cytolytic killing of virus-infected cells*' is defined as cytolysis of SC-2-infected target host cells by MHC (Major Histocompatibility Complex class I -unrestricted cytotoxic lymphocytes (CTLs as a result of enhanced uptake of pNAb-complexed progeny virions into tissue-resident APCs. Cytolysis of SC-2-infected target host cells mediates recovery from C-19 disease.

For the purpose of this manuscript, SC-2 variants that are **more infectious and highly virulent** have the capacity to provoke *'Ab-independent enhancement of severe C-19 disease' (AIESD)*.

Cognate and Noncognate T Help

It is well known that induction of memory B cells relies on physical contact between T helper and B cells. Assistance provided by these T cells (called 'T help'; Th) can either be cognate or noncognate.

'Cognate' refers to a direct, cell-cell interaction between a B cell and the reactive T cell that is based upon specific recognition of B cell (Bc) peptide epitopes that are conjugated to an antigenic peptide presented within MHC class II and recognized by the antigen(Ag)-specific receptor of the reactive T cell.

'Noncognate' refers to a direct, cell-cell interaction between a B cell and the reactive T cell that is based upon specific recognition of Bc peptide epitopes facilitated by *bystander MHC class II-restricted CD4+ T helper* cells. Bystander MHC class II-restricted CD4+ T helper cells are activated by MHC class II-binding peptides other than those conjugated to the specific Bc target epitope. By providing *noncognate* T help, activated bystander Th cells can therefore allow immune recognition of specific Bc epitopes that are not juxtaposed to a Th antigen.

Bc epitopes that receive T help from noncognate (i.e., bystander) Th cells or that are subdominant induce low-affinity Abs. Although *immune subdominant Bc epitopes* receive T help from cognate Th cells, the provided T help is weak as subdominant Bc epitopes are outcompeted by *immunodominant Bc epitopes* for assistance from CD4+ Th cells. Whereas strong T help allows for priming of high-affinity memory B cells (i.e., endowed with B cell receptors [BCRs] that bind with high affinity to their epitopes), weak T help provided by noncognate T help or to subdominant Bc epitopes will result in priming of low-affinity memory B cells (i.e., endowed with BCRs that have low affinity for their epitopes).

Weaker immunogenicity is usually rooted in a higher level of evolutionary epitope conservation. This explains why subdominant and noncognate Th-dependent Ags induce Ag-specific, low-affinity memory B cells that secrete *broadly* functional Abs.

Lastly, Bc epitopes that are completely *Th-independent* (i.e., they do not receive any type of T help[3] are not normally immunogenic and called 'immunocryptic'[4]. Provided these motifs present as repetitive polymeric patterns,[5] they can still elicit Abs. However, due to lack of T help assistance to the activated B cells, these Abs are short-lived and have very weak affinity. They are therefore poorly specific (or 'multi-/polyspecific') and nonfunctional (i.e., devoid of neutralizing capacity.

References

Please find references associated with this book in support of my hypothesis online at https://www.voiceforscienceandsolidarity.org/blog/resources-accompanying-my-book or by scanning this QR Code.

Important Note to the Reader

For the purpose of this manuscript, unless otherwise explicitly stated, all instances of 'vaccine' or 'vaccines' refer to C-19 vaccines. Similarly, discussion of vaccinated or not vaccinated individuals refers to C-19 vaccination unless otherwise made explicit. Discussion of infection, exposure and variants refers to that which is due to SC-2 whereas discussion of disease, hospitalization and mortality refers to that which is due to C-19.

Discussion of the pandemic relates to both C-19 and SC-2 because the term 'pandemic' applies to both the infection as well as the disease caused by the infection.

Table of Contents

1.2.7. PNNAb-dependent VBTIs enable highly vaccinated populations to rapidly re-orient cognate Th-dependent immune pressure on variable S-associated epitopes to noncognate Th-dependent immune pressure on more conserved S-associated epitopes. Subsequent Ab-independent VBTIs allow re-orientation of noncognate Th-dependent immune pressure on more conserved S-associated epitopes to Th-independent immune pressure on a highly conserved S-NTD-associated antigenic determinant. This evolution allows PNNAb-dependent or (PNN)Ab-independent VBTIs to cause fast and large-scale viral immune escape. 20

1.2.8. Rapid immune escape from refocused humoral immune responses elicited by VBTIs with Omicron relies on *convergent devolution* of a limited subset of more conserved S-NTD or S-RBD domains to antigenic determinants that are derived from the ancestral Wuhan-Hu lineage or pre-Omicron variants, respectively. 23

1.2.9. To maximize the effect on viral immune escape, SIR-1–following VBTIs with OOV–had to precede SIR-2. 26

1.2.10. Once highly infectious Omicron descendants circulate, neither additional vaccination (e.g., additional booster doses or vaccination of additional age groups such as children) nor a complete halt of the mass vaccination program will be able to prevent highly vaccinated populations from increasing immune pressure on viral virulence. 28

1.2.11. It is impossible to understand the disastrous evolution of this immune escape pandemic without understanding SIR, i.e., without an understanding of how Omicron and mRNA-based vaccinations reshaped the affinity and breadth of the humoral anti-S response in vaccinated individuals. 31

populations to a *single* event of *gradually* increasing immune pressure that will take *some time* to *sequentially select* a *single highly virulent* variant (HIVICRON). 60

Chapter Five

Research on the immune escape pandemic has become an exercise in mutational stamp collection that does not yield any concrete predictions on the societal impact. Instead, immunological ignorance and mainstream narratives prevail.

highly vaccinated countries, yet several scientists continue to pretend that the situation is under control and that protection against severe disease is durable and largely relies on cross-reactive memory T cells.   86

5.6. The scientific community agrees that convergent evolution of 'concerning' immune escape variants in highly vaccinated populations results from population-level immune selection pressure placed on the virus. Why does no one investigate the origin of this population-level immune pressure?   89

Chapter Six   90

Even if the road is bumpy, a naturally trained CBIIS is the (only) key to protection from viral immune escape variants and to taming a viral immune escape pandemic.   **90**

6.1. In contrast to vaccine-primed immunity, adaptive immune priming by natural infection is dampened by the CBIIS. Vaccinated individuals acquired protection from disease caused by pre-Omicron through vaccine-induced NAbs whereas the unvaccinated acquired such protection through a combination of trained CBIIS and NAbs. However, this immune protection did not suffice to protect either group from BTIs with Omicron. However, trained CBII in the unvaccinated prevented these BTIs from enabling SIR.   91

6.2. Enhanced intrinsic infectiousness of immune escape variants diminishes viral shedding. As viral infectiousness of newly emerging (more virulent) immune escape variants does no longer increase, trained CBII in the unvaccinated can catch up with new emerging variants to protect the unvaccinated from symptomatic infection. Sterilizing immunity in the unvaccinated combined with a high mortality rate in the vaccinated will eventually lead to natural extinction of the pandemic in highly vaccinated populations.   96

The Inescapable Immune Escape Pandemic

Nobody Can Conceal The Science
That Nature Is Now Desperate To Unveil

Society In Highly Vaccinated Countries
Will Be Caught By Surprise

Prologue

From the moment I heard about the intention to "mass vaccinate" people, I knew that it would lead to viral immune escape and have disastrous consequences. Others, regardless of their professional or educational backgrounds, felt the same way based on their innate "common sense", but couldn't explain why they felt something was fundamentally wrong. They were left to argue against the idea using arguments about side effects. I felt a strong urge to reveal the truth on this topic - I knew from the start that my understanding was correct. Knowing that I was right motivated me even more.

I have had a long-standing career in several different disciplines that I've tried to synergize in order to understand the complex interactions between pathogens and the immune system: immunology, virology, vaccinology, and evolutionary biology. Each of these disciplines has its own "rules". To "connect the dots", one must first respect many rules... and, as it turns out, the concept of mass vaccination violates all of them! Nature has shaped the rules of these biological disciplines over thousands of years, whereas the "rules" of technology are man-made and only apply when validated by biology (e.g., aircraft technology must be validated by the laws of gravity), and not the other way around.

I have always had a passion for the life sciences. Since life, or nature, always tells the truth, I am passionate about sharing these truths I have discovered from my favorite scientific fields. But how does one discover the truth? I knew I had to be very critical and open to all questions. I knew I couldn't leave any stone unturned. I knew I couldn't rest until I had put all the pieces of the puzzle together. I knew I wouldn't discover the truth until I saw the forest and not just the trees.

However, I realized that passion for the truth and searching for it wasn't sufficient. Somebody needed to document the truth and warn the world. I felt compelled to undertake this task because my diversified and professional experience in this field has given me credibility. And also because I was independent. I knew I needed to react. I would never have tolerated anyone arguing that the current "health emergency" was unpredictable; that it was unprecedented and therefore all health authorities worldwide had done their very best, based upon the knowledge that was available. I want the world to know that nothing is more predictable than the disastrous consequences resulting from mankind's massive intervention in the delicate ecosystem governing pathogen-immune system interactions. That it was entirely predictable, from the very start of this massive "experiment", that this would cause Nature to take an unprecedented toll on human lives. I also want the world to know that those who decided to conduct this reckless experiment on the entire human species have been repeatedly warned, but have chosen not to listen. They have, instead, chosen to put their egos, money, arrogance and political ambitions above dignity and respect for humanity and nature.

I knew I had the key to the truth, and needed to open people's eyes to allow that truth to expose the stupidity of those who, despite having no understanding and even less respect for biology or the laws of Nature, foolishly believed they could control it; to allow the truth to show them the sophistication of Nature, as opposed to the futility of technologies which attempt, but will never succeed, in breaking her rules. How far will they go before grasping the simple concept that even the most innovative technology cannot override and control the natural forces and concepts of biology?

Another key reason for writing this book is to protect the children. I care about our children, grandchildren, and future generations in general. Even though I am aware that man rarely learns from the past, I want to remind them that the happiness and success of our species depends on our harmonious coexistence with Nature. This equilibrium - whose complexity may be difficult for some of us to understand and, probably for others, impossible to accept - should not be disturbed by man-made interventions that Nature does not recognize as her own, and with her power will thwart every time. It is therefore critical that we attempt to understand and respect her complexity before massively intervening with technologies that possibly violate her laws, as there can be no doubt that Nature knows how to remind us of the force of her will and her power.

I hope to be an example to the next generation and encourage them to always have a critical but open mind and to strive for the truth. The truth may not always bring peace of mind, especially for those who prefer to erase it, escape it, alter or abolish it, but it will always be a faithful ally to those who seek it, trust in it, and live by it. There is no gray zone when it comes to the truth. It's a clear-cut choice that each one of us must make every day.

On a positive note, I am strongly convinced that our children will have the opportunity to build a better world once this crisis is over. I want them to know that the world will need them to serve as architects of a new society, founded on humility, dignity, integrity, and a sense of community. This, I believe, is the only way to make humanity great again!

Foreword

Three years into the course of the COVID-19 pandemic, there is a lot of confusion, much polarization, and there are many questions.

Why has the pandemic continued for so long?

Why are we seeing one new variant after another?

Why is each new variant more infectious and more vaccine-resistant than its predecessors?

Why are fully vaccinated and boosted people becoming reinfected, repeatedly?

Is the COVID mass vaccination campaign itself responsible for the above, by causing "immune escape" phenomena? Or is the main problem that not enough people are vaccinated and/or boosted with the currently available COVID-19 vaccines?

On balance, at both an individual level and a population level, has the COVID-19 mass vaccination campaign been wise? Or is it threatening Humanity?

Is it safe, necessary, and wise to be injecting the current COVID-19 vaccines into infants, toddlers, older children, adolescents, and young adults?

What is going to happen? Is the pandemic subsiding and heading into a harmless endemic phase? Or is the mass vaccination campaign transforming the pandemic into a prolonged and potentially disastrous "immune escape" pandemic?

Should the COVID-19 mass vaccination campaign be continued, even escalated? Or should the campaign be immediately halted?

What are the scientific truths? Why is there so much controversy? Whose opinions are more scientifically sound; the promoters of the mass vaccination campaign or the scientists and physicians who have challenged the scientific merits and wisdom of that campaign?

Whom should the public trust? Why has there not been more open dialogue?

In this book, Dr. Geert Vanden Bossche addresses the above questions by delving deeply into the complex science involved. He has written a brilliant and invaluable scientific treatise regarding the dynamic interplay between the immune system and viruses, how that interplay is affected by the COVID-19 mass vaccination campaign, and what consequences can be anticipated.

Dr. Vanden Bossche reminds us that the immune system is an extraordinarily complex and ingenious ecosystem. It is a collaborative network comprised of many diverse components, each with its own highly valued aptitudes. It is conservative, revolutionary, and radical all at the same time. It is constantly engaged in complex, carefully-balanced interactions with viruses and other pathogens. It has developed and perfected its capabilities over a period of hundreds of thousands of years. Humanity owes its very existence to the marvelous immune system.

As powerful, intelligent, and flexible as our immune system is, it is nevertheless delicate. In that sense the immune ecosystem is as fragile as any other ecosystem in nature. Just as we need to protect other natural ecosystems (e.g. wetlands, rainforests, etc.) from misguided human interventions, we need to protect the human ecosystem from misguided human interventions. Any interference with the immune system's perfected capacities and delicate balances must be carefully thought out and based on a deep understanding of the science involved---particularly the evolutionary dynamics associated with the complex interactions between the immune system, pathogens (e.g., viruses, and vaccines.

All of us, particularly the scientists, physicians, and other health professionals who are playing roles in the COVID-19 response, must appreciate the complexity of the immune ecosystem and how ill-advised interventions, even if well-intended, can have disastrous consequences. Indeed, the COVID-19 pandemic cannot be properly understood and managed without a deep understanding of the immunology, virology, vaccinology, evolutionary biology, and glycosylation biology involved---without a deep appreciation of the dynamic interplay between the immune system, viruses, and vaccines, at both a population level and an individual level.

Throughout the COVID-19 pandemic, Dr. Vanden Bossche has been the leading voice regarding appreciation of the complexity and genius of the immune ecosystem and the consequences of unwise manipulation of it.

I first became aware of Dr. Vanden Bossche in April 2021 when I watched and listened to him being interviewed by Dr. Philip McMillan, a physician in the UK. During that interview Dr. Vanden Bossche explained his strictly science-based concerns about predictable deleterious effects of the COVID-19 mass vaccination campaign. As I watched and listened, it became clear that Dr Vanden Bossche had an extraordinarily deep understanding of the immunology, virology, vaccinology, evolutionary biology, and glycosylation biology involved. He has had extensive experience with the development and testing of vaccines, including recognition and understanding of vaccine successes and vaccine failures and the dangers of certain vaccination approaches. He understands the potential consequences of an ill-advised mass vaccination campaign on a population level, not just on an individual level. It was clear that he applies a rigorous multidisciplinary scientific approach and sees connections that others may not see. It was evident that he had uncommon insight regarding the science involved in the COVID-19 situation.

In addition to his extensive scientific expertise, and of equal or more importance, the strength of his character was clearly evident. As I watched and listened, I sensed that his motivations were pure; that he was honest, altruistic, disciplined, and doggedly determined to seek the most accurate scientific understanding of the COVID-19 situation and share it with the scientific community and the general public, for Humanity's sake, not for his own sake. I sensed great ethical integrity as well as great scientific integrity. Both are essential, particularly in science and medicine.

It was evident that he was deeply concerned about the consequences of what he viewed as an misguided COVID-19 mass vaccination campaign, and that his concerns were strictly based on science, not on any other agenda. It was clear that he is not "anti-vaccination;" he is only against scientifically and ethically unsound vaccination campaigns. His explanations made scientific sense to me. I concluded that his hypotheses and concerns should be the top issues for discussion, among scientists and physicians and within the public.

So, what are his understandings and specific concerns? As he explained in the above- mentioned interview and has extensively detailed in this book, his main messages are as follows:

> It is unwise to try to end an active, ongoing pandemic, like the COVID-19 pandemic, by implementing, in the midst of that pandemic, a mass vaccination campaign (across all age groups) that uses vaccines (like the COVID-19 vaccines) that do not adequately prevent infection or transmission of the virus, do not produce sterilizing immunity, and, thereby, do not contribute to herd immunity.

As Dr. Vanden Bossche explains, in great scientific detail, such a mass vaccination campaign predictably results in a prolonged series of dominant SARS-CoV-2 variants, each becoming more infectious and more vaccine-resistant than its predecessors; and is highly likely to result, eventually, in the emergence of an SARS-CoV-2 variant that is more virulent than all predecessors. This is due to the predictable natural selection of viral variants that are able to "escape" the intense immune pressures placed on the virus at a population level by the COVID- 19 mass vaccination campaign. The result is a prolonged "immune escape" pandemic. Furthermore, Dr. Vanden Bossche warns that, by side-lining the innate immune system, the COVID-19 vaccines harmfully interfere with normal immune education and function (particularly of NK cells, especially when given to young children. As a pediatrician, I particularly appreciate Dr. Vanden Bossche's warning that the COVID-19 vaccines interfere with the foundational education (and subsequent ongoing training of a young child's innate immune system and, thereby, predispose children to autoimmunity, malignancy, and difficulty handling other glycosylated viruses. These same predisposing effects apply to older children and adults.

Not only did Dr. Vanden Bossche appropriately predict these consequences of the COVID-19 mass vaccination campaign, but his predictions have also turned out to be accurate. Dominant SARS-CoV-2 variants have become increasingly infectious and increasingly resistant to vaccines; recent variants have been shown to be more virulent in vitro; and there is legitimate concern that new variants will soon become more virulent in vivo. Furthermore, there is clear evidence that the vaccines are undermining and harming normal immune function. As Dr, Vanden Bossche explains, these problems are due to the COVID-19 mass vaccination campaign, not to lack of citizen participation in that campaign.

Dr. Vanden Bossche goes on to explain that once a more virulent, more infectious, and more vaccine-resistant variant becomes dominant, the consequences for Humanity could be catastrophic. As he predicted, the vaccination campaign has prolonged the pandemic and made it more dangerous. The sobering conclusion is that, in the final analysis, more lives will have been lost, cumulatively (over the past 3 years and in the many months ahead, because of the COVID-19 mass vaccination campaign than would have been lost if we had never implemented that mass vaccination campaign and had relied, instead, on the competency of the immune system and on selective vaccination of the elderly and otherwise vulnerable (but only if a vaccine with proven safety and efficacy were available). Dr. Vanden Bossche's conclusion is that the COVID-19 mass vaccination campaign must be halted immediately, before more harm is done.

The above understandings and concerns obviously conflict with the message provided by the promoters of the prevailing COVID-19 narrative and its mass vaccination campaign, a message that the COVID-19 vaccines are: remarkably "safe and effective"; they "save lives"; and, "get vaccinated; it's your social duty."

Promoters of the mass vaccination campaign have ignored Dr. Vanden Bossche's understandings and warnings. Their response to his concerns and scientific explanations has been silence.

Unfortunately, healthy, respectful, scientific dialogue between promoters of the mass vaccination campaign and scientists/physicians who appreciate Dr. Vanden Bossche's concerns has not occurred, despite the great efforts of the challengers to engage the promoters in such dialogue. Only one narrative has been allowed---the "get vaccinated and get boosted" narrative. Thoughtful, knowledgeable, caring physicians who have challenged the scientific merits of the COVID-19 mass vaccination campaign have been censored, demonized, accused of spreading harmful misinformation/disinformation, and have been threatened with loss of their medical licenses. Some have had their medical licenses indefinitely suspended.

A fundamental principle of science and medicine is engagement in scientific dialogue and encouragement of challenges to prevailing thinking. This principle is violated when promoters of the prevailing COVID-19 narrative forbid challenges and refuse to engage in scientific dialogue. The resultant lack of healthy scientific dialogue has slowed advancement of knowledge and has caused confusion and ugly polarization that has ripped communities apart-- -health care communities, society as a whole, even families.

The public, including physicians and health professionals, desperately needs and deserves help in understanding the scientific complexity of the COVID-19 situation and the controversies involved. The public needs and deserves to receive information from a scientist who is not only deeply knowledgeable, but also altruistic, honest, properly motivated, and without conflict of interest.

In my view, Dr. Vanden Bossche's scientific treatise is the most important analysis that has been written during the COVID-19 pandemic. This book can and should be read not only by scientists, physicians, and public health policymakers, but also by politicians and citizens who have a limited science background. It is not important for the reader to necessarily master the extraordinarily complex information Dr. Vanden Bossche provides. What is important is to develop a solid general impression of how complex, ingenious, marvelous, and, yet, delicate and fragile the immune ecosystem is and how careful and responsible we must be when we manipulate it. This book will help its readers to appreciate these complexities and share new insights with others.

This book provides scientifically sound information that will help demystify the COVID situation and can serve as the substance for much needed open dialogue---within scientific communities, within the public at large, and within families. This book has the potential to bring people together; facilitate respectful conversation; elevate understanding; reduce confusion, polarization, and intolerance; and help heal rifts. It will help Humanity to properly manage this pandemic and make certain that mistakes are not repeated in the future. It will help us to correct current misguided arrangements and create new arrangements that will respect and protect the precious human immune ecosystem and honor fundamental principles of science, medicine, and ethics.

Robert Rennebohm, MD
January, 2023

Summary

As a first line of immune defense, the cell-based innate immune system (CBIIS) is critically important for removal of most of the SARS-CoV-2 (SC-2) viral load upon primary infection and subsequent re-infection (as titers of infection-primed antibodies decline quite rapidly). Training of the CBIIS (i.e., comprising adaptation and functional reprogramming of innate Natural Killer [NK] cells via epigenetic imprinting) may sometimes even obviate the need for engaging the adaptive immune system.

Population-level immune pressure on viral infectiousness following mass vaccination with S(pike) protein-based vaccines during the pandemic eventually caused SC-2 to sideline this vitally important first line of immune defense. As large scale suboptimal humoral immune pressure on viral infectiousness eventually drove natural selection and expansion of an immune escape variant (i.e., Omicron) that vaccine-induced antibodies (Abs) could no longer sufficiently neutralize, infection-enhancing *polyreactive non-neutralizing Abs* (PNNAbs) came into effect and caused PNNAb-dependent enhancement of viral infectiousness. OOV (original Omicron variant) and its early subvariants (i.e., early Omicron-derived subvariants; EOSVs) became the first lineages that managed to provoke large-scale PNNAb-dependent breakthrough infections in highly vaccinated populations.

PNNAb-dependent breakthrough infections in vaccinees (VBTIs) enable sidelining of the CBIIS and are responsible for steric immune refocusing (SIR), a phenomenon which occurs when anti-S Abs bind with low affinity to newly synthesized S protein and thereby sterically mask the immunodominant S-associated epitopes. SIR therefore forces the immune system to focus on co-localized subdominant epitopes. By seeking noncognate T help from recalled, previously vaccine-induced CD4+ T memory cells, these immune subdominant epitopes prime new, broadly functional Abs targeting S-associated antigenic domains that are more conserved, but less immunogenic.

Because these new, broadly functional Abs enabled vaccinated individuals to prevent productive infection and thereby paused viral transmission and immune escape, I have underestimated the time it would take for new, highly infectious and potentially virulent variants to emerge. However, these Abs have only short-lived neutralizing or infection-inhibiting capacity and take several months to mature. Therefore, protection against productive infection conferred by SIR-enabling VBTIs (and SIR-enabling mRNA boosters, and hence, the slowdown immune escape experienced, has also been short-lived. Because of their low affinity, these broadly functional Abs rapidly exerted high immune pressure on the targeted conserved epitopes which eventually precipitated *large-scale* viral immune escape.

My analysis unambiguously proves that the mass vaccination experiment has been responsible for selecting and promoting dominant propagation of Omicron in highly vaccinated populations. Whereas '*original antigenic sin*' has been driving immune escape during the pre-Omicron phase of the pandemic in all countries conducting mass vaccination campaigns, '*SIR*' has been responsible for the spectacular evolutionary dynamics of this *immune escape pandemic* once Omicron dominantly circulated. As Omicron caused SIR-enabling VBTIs and as SIR caused highly vaccinated populations to exert high immune pressure on more conserved, subdominant S-associated domains, natural selection and dominant propagation of Omicron has been required and sufficient to drive *large scale* viral immune escape.

Continuation of the mass vaccination program during the Omicron phase of the pandemic has only expedited the selectional adaptive evolution of the virus as booster doses and growing vaccine coverage rates allowed for more frequent and widespread SIR-enabling VBTIs. *mRNA-based* vaccines in particular have dramatically accelerated the immune escape dynamics of SC-2 as— in contrast to the other, non-mRNA-based vaccines—they elicit low-affinity anti-S Abs[6] directed at S protein that is expressed on the surface of the mRNA-transfected host cells.

By way of *steric masking*, these low-affinity Abs silence S-associated immunodominant epitopes expressed on the surface of free-circulating S protein once the latter is released from the mRNA-transfected cells, or once progeny virus is released from infected

l

host cells. mRNA-based vaccines are therefore *SIR-enabling in their own right* and promote the occurrence of PNNAb-dependent VBTIs. SIR causes SC-2 to irreversibly sideline the CBIIS and inevitably drives vaccines to exert large-scale immune pressure on viral infectiousness. The resulting immune escape mutations eventually converged to the receptor-binding domain of spike protein (S-RBD) to confer a high-level of intrinsic viral infectiousness to the currently co-circulating Omicron descendants.

Because of their high intrinsic infectiousness, these new emerging Omicron descendants provoke a high incidence of Ab-independent VBTIs in highly vaccinated populations. However, as the production of PNNAbs is now no longer keeping pace with enhanced adsorption of highly infectious progeny virus onto migratory *dendritic cells* (DCs), PNNAb-mediated population-level immune pressure on viral *trans* infectiousness is gradually increasing upon (re-)exposure of vaccinated individuals to these highly infectious Omicron descendants. At the same time, diminished concentration of free progeny SC-2 virions allows for their binding to a relatively higher concentration of pre-existing, potentially neutralizing vaccine-induced Abs (pNAbs). As the latter facilitate virus uptake into patrolling antigen (Ag)-presenting cells (APCs), *Ab-independent* VBTIs result in enhanced uptake of SC-2 virions into APCs, and therefore enhance activation of MHC class I-unrestricted CTLs (cytolytic T lymphocytes) that eliminate virus-infected cells. Consequently, high intrinsic infectiousness of currently co-circulating variants is thought to gradually increase PNNAb-dependent immune pressure on viral *trans* infectiousness[7] while diminishing shedding and attenuating disease symptoms.

Consequently, enhanced killing of virus-infected cells is inseparably connected with enhanced PNNAb-mediated immune pressure on viral *trans* infectiousness/virulence. At a large scale, this gradually increasing immune pressure on viral virulence is now promoting natural selection of variants that have picked up mutations[8] allowing them to overcome PNNAb-mediated inhibition of viral *trans* infectiousness/virulence, which is the final mechanism of vaccine-mediated adaptive immune defense still currently protecting vaccinated individuals against severe disease. As more and more highly vaccinated populations are currently witnessing co-circulation of more infectious Omicron descendants, we are facing a health emergency of international concern.

As a first step towards breaching the virulence-neutralizing capacity of PNNAbs, antigenically distinct Omicron descendants that pair enhanced infectiousness with enhanced virulence may be selected in distinct highly vaccinated populations to dominantly spread. Given the highly conserved nature of the PNNAb-binding site within S-NTD, it is likely that such dominant lineages (e.g., XBB.1.5. will evolve the same O-glycosite mutation to abrogate large-scale immune pressure on viral virulence when the latter has grown to a critical threshold. Asynchronous selection of such highly virulent variants is likely to provoke separate, rapidly rising waves of Ab-independent enhancement of severe disease (AIESD in those populations.

This evolution would undoubtedly put the lives of many vaccinated individuals with poorly trained cell-based innate immunity (CBII) at high risk. However, as the vast majority of the unvaccinated have by now sufficiently trained their CBIIS to control productive infection of highly infectious variants, there is a strong rationale to believe that they will not only be spared from AIESD but even from disease altogether.

mRNA vaccines likely trigger immune refocusing as of the first injection following productive infection or as a booster following primary vaccination, or as of the first productive infection following a primary series of mRNA vaccinations. Because of this, large scale deployment of mRNA-based vaccines is not only likely to have expedited immune escape but also to have largely prevented or abrogated training of the CBIIS by natural infection. Based on immunological considerations and a multitude of serological and epidemiological data from the literature, it seems undeniable that usage of mRNA vaccines has significantly contributed to accelerating the tragic evolution of this immune escape pandemic.

As exposure to OOV or EOSVs could trigger symptomatic PNNAb-mediated BTIs in vaccinated individuals regardless of the training status of their CBIIS, the occurrence of symptomatic infection with Omicron does not inform whether the PNNAb-mediated BTI enabled SIR and therefore resulted in irrevocable sidelining of their CBIIS. However, SIR-enabling VBTIs have a poor prognosis for both individual and public health due to inhibition of cell-based innate immune training and large-scale immune escape, respectively. Unfortunately, there is currently no validated assay that allows for a reliable measure of the level of cell-based innate immune memory.

Given that both mRNA-based vaccines and high titers of poorly neutralizing Abs in vaccinated individuals promote or trigger SIR-enabling VBTIs (which sideline the CBIIS), it is fair to conclude that only a few categories of vaccinated individuals are likely to have a CBIIS that can be sufficiently trained to protect them from more infectious and virulent variants to the same extent as the unvaccinated. These include:

> *All healthy vaccinees who had only received a single injection of an mRNA-based vaccine or no more than 2 injections with a non-mRNA-based vaccine prior to developing symptomatic VBTI and who refrained from booster shots after said symptomatic VBTI.*

It is equally difficult to fathom that our leading scientists and public health experts believe that infections with Omicron and its descendants are a blessing due to their pairing of a high level of viral infectiousness with mild pathogenic properties (and as side effects are largely denied, anyway). However, if they truly believe this will enable highly vaccinated populations to build herd immunity and drive SC-2 into endemicity, their narrative is not only an unforgivable insult to the science but also a profoundly unethical and despicable blow to the face of all those who have been coerced into vaccination by their employers, governments, health authorities, educational institutions or other influential bodies.

Introduction

Given the rapid evolution of the virus, I have had no choice but to write up my analysis in a hurry. You may know of other relevant aspects not covered in this text, deplore some lack of fine-tuning, or you may even find inaccuracies, but I am sure immunologists and vaccinologists will grasp the alarming message. Some chapters may be partially redundant—I had no time to eliminate these redundancies, but I don't think they pose a problem to the reader. On the contrary, a different phrasing of the same concept/mechanism might contribute to a better understanding of the complex interactions at play. As the virus has been evolving rapidly and the evolutionary dynamics of the immune response have continuously been changing as well, I have sometimes used the present tense and at other times the past tense or even the past perfect/completed past tense.

The sequence and titles of chapters have not been chosen to serve an educational purpose, as in a regular textbook, but rather to focus and elaborate on clear-cut statements, remarkable observations and relevant but unanswered questions related to the current immune escape pandemic.

In my analysis, I am not concentrating on the nomenclature and mutational specifics of new emerging SARS-CoV-2 (SC-2) immune escape [sub]variants but on changes to the population-level immune pressure underlying key antigenic changes of these variants. As data from viral, biological and clinical analyses gathered during this pandemic have been rapidly evolving, I have tried to capitalize on the overall evolutionary dynamics of these data rather than on specific snapshots thereof.

The purpose of my analysis has therefore been to describe the scientific rationale underlying the evolutionary dynamics of this immune escape pandemic and to demonstrate that its complexity is rooted in both the evolving host immune pressure placed on the virus and the adaptation of the virus to this immune pressure. My investigation aims at proving that none of the observed viral immune escape is coincidental, but rather results from evolving large scale immune pressure caused initially by the mass vaccination program, and since the advent of Omicron has evolved into a self-catalyzing chain of enhanced immune escape.

The current contribution builds on my previous analysis from May 9th, 2022 (entitled: *Poor virus-neutralizing capacity in highly vaccinated populations could soon lead to a fulminant spread of SARS-CoV-2 super variants that are highly infectious and highly virulent in vaccinated individuals while being fully resistant to all existing and future spike-based vaccines (ref. 5)*). It may be important to consult this earlier contribution as I am regularly referring to important drivers of the immunopathogenesis of severe disease (e.g., viral *trans* infectiousness and *trans* fusion and their correlation with syncytia formation or inhibition thereof by S protein-associated O-glycosite mutations) that I have explained in great detail.

Based on this previous analysis, *I had already predicted that the mass vaccination experiment would drive the emergence of highly infectious variants that would also prove to increase their virulence as a result of increasing immune pressure on viral trans infectiousness.* Although my predictions on the evolutionary dynamics of SC-2 and the immunological mechanisms underlying the immune escape still fully apply, the timeline I had predicted for these highly problematic variants to emerge was not correct. In my current report, I am explaining why the timeline I previously proposed (QIII 2022) was too short. Back then, I did not realize that SC-2 would need to further increase its intrinsic infectiousness to cause highly vaccinated populations to exert increasing immune pressure on viral virulence. In order to do so, Omicron first had to provoke widespread vaccine breakthrough infections (VBTIs), as those were paramount to trigger steric immune refocusing (SIR). SIR enables the host immune system to expedite immune escape by placing high immune pressure on more conserved S(pike)-associated domains that induce broadly functional but short-lived Abs. As the latter allowed for a temporary decrease in viral infection and transmission, viral immune escape dynamics (and hence, the timeline I anticipated) were delayed.

I also further explain the immunological mechanisms involved in SIR and how they are triggered by VBTIs as well as mRNA-based vaccines. I'll also dive into why and how co-circulation of highly infectious Omicron descendants are currently improving cell-based *innate* immune function in the vast majority of the unvaccinated while improving cell-based *adaptive* immune protection against disease symptoms and SC-2 shedding in the vaccinated. As improved protection in vaccinated individuals is inextricably linked to enhanced immune pressure on viral virulence, and as the latter is likely to drive the emergence of new, dominantly propagating variants capable of triggering Ab-independent enhancement of severe disease (AIESD), *I am warning highly vaccinated societies that they will be caught by surprise.*

Together with my previous contribution (ref. 5), the present work aims to unambiguously document the scientific plausibility of an imminent public health disaster and to provide compelling evidence of how and why the mass vaccination program has been driving this pandemic into disastrous immune escape instead of endemicity. My own multidisciplinary insights combined with the relevant observations reported in the non-exhaustive list of publications attached at the end of this book should be more than sufficient to understand and predict the evolutionary dynamics of viral immune escape in highly vaccinated populations.

As mentioned before, my scientific approach to understanding the evolutionary dynamics of this immune escape pandemic has been based upon deductive reasoning and holistic assessment. There is, in my opinion, no other rational method to analyze biological phenomena with such a high level of interdisciplinary complexity than the findings I've included in this book.

To validate the conclusions of my work, there is likely no better citation than that of Sherlock-Holmes. *"How often have I said to you that when you have eliminated the impossible, whatever remains, however improbable, must be the truth?"*

As a result, a theory has been developed that is not only consistent with the current clinical and epidemiological observations, but which is also supported by scientifically validated principles. This theory is now translating to extremely concerning predictions about the potential implications of the ongoing mass vaccination program on both individual and public health. *As the conclusions make perfect scientific sense, its predictive value should be taken very seriously.*

However, my predictions are a type of science that is not recognized by our traditional schools of thought. It is therefore the type that no scientific journal may be willing to publish. Our academic institutions and scientific media are (willfully?) blinded by their atomistic approaches which prevent them from seeing the forest for the trees. The depth of my analysis of this pandemic sharply contrasts with the simplicity and shallowness of the mainstream narrative key opinion leaders, whom scientific experts seemingly support; it shows how profoundly their scientific mindset is perverted by conflicts of interest. No matter how high they are, their ivory towers are merely breeding grounds for silo thinking. It is no wonder their inhabitants will never understand how the mass vaccination experiment turned this pandemic into the largest and most dangerous gain-of-function experiment ever conducted in the history of biology. If they were to read this book, I cannot imagine they would not change their minds. Unfortunately, I doubt they have the appetite to do so.

For regular updates, please visit Voice For Science and Solidarity, which you may locate online at https://www.voiceforscienceandsolidarity.org/or by scanning the code below.

Chapter One

Omicron! What have you done?!

1.1.Exposure of vaccinated individuals to Omicron puts immune mechanisms at work that are fundamentally different from those elicited in the unvaccinated. Whereas Omicron diminished the protective capacity in the former and promoted its own immune escape, it strengthened protection in the latter without driving immune escape.

This statement may be puzzling to our experts and health authorities. According to their interpretation, humoral immune protection against infection or disease provided by Abs naturally-induced in the unvaccinated due to previous productive infection are short-lived and therefore unable to provide a level of protection as good as that conferred by vaccine-induced (i.e., anti-Wuhan-Hu S) Abs. This is because they still don't seem to understand the critical role of trained CBII in removing the bulk of viral load upon subsequent exposure. Since a trained CBIIS kills virus-infected host cells at an early stage of infection, uptake of free circulating virus by APCs is relatively low and adaptive immune priming is therefore weak. This sharply contrasts with immunization by vaccines, all of which are non-replicating. The vaccines therefore do not train the CBIIS whereas they strongly stimulate the adaptive immune system. Consequently, naturally induced anti-S Abs do not last as long as vaccine-induced anti-S Abs.

  After previously protecting against disease from pre-Omicron variants, the immune mechanisms at play in vaccinated individuals are – for now – still largely efficient against all Omicron (sub)variant(s) in terms of protection against (severe) disease [9]. Although the evolving protective immune mechanisms at play in vaccinated individuals comprise several adaptive immune effectors, none of them is sufficiently functional because of inadequate or deficient immunological memory[10] (i.e., *noncognate* Th-dependent broadly neutralizing or infection-inhibiting Abs, *Th-independent* PNNAbs and *Th-independent* MHC class I-unrestricted CTLs). The vast majority of vaccinated individuals are still largely protected from (severe) disease thanks to *trans* infection-inhibiting PNNAbs still present in sufficiently high concentrations, and enhanced activation of MHC class I-unrestricted CTLs (chapters 3.1. and 3.3.) (fig. 11). But the clock is ticking as large-scale, PNNAb-mediated immune pressure on viral virulence is steadily increasing. The devastating health impact of a new and highly infectious variant that will have acquired a high level of intrinsic *trans* infectiousness and hence, capable of triggering PNNAb-dependent enhancement of severe disease, is imminent.

Whereas during the pre-Omicron phase of the pandemic, protection of frail people (i.e., the elderly and those with co-morbidities or otherwise immune suppressed) against disease was clearly superior in vaccinated individuals as compared to the non-vaccinated, the vast majority of unvaccinated persons became increasingly well protected against disease symptoms after previous infection(s) trained their CBII[11]. The CBIIS has sterilizing capacity towards infected cells, irrespective of the antigenic properties of the variant. Strong reduction of viral load combined with rapidly waning titers of anti-S Abs (both due to a properly trained CBIIS) explain why the unvaccinated (at least those who did not fully isolate themselves during the pre-Omicron phase), but not the vaccinated, managed to prevent SIR-enabling BTIs upon their exposure to Omicron (figs. 5 and 7). In contrast to the vaccinated, the unvaccinated therefore neither drove immune escape during the pre-Omicron phase nor after Omicron emerged.

1.2. mRNA vaccines and Omicron-mediated VBTIs trigger SIR and have therefore been throwing more oil on the immune escape fire.[12]

1.2.1. Pre- or post-infection vaccination with mRNA-based vaccines is a major driver of SIR.

Provided an antigen is simultaneously presented to the immune system in different formats, primed T helper cells can provide both cognate and noncognate T help to the same Ag (e.g., S protein in the case of SC-2) and thereby elicit Ag-specific Abs with high and low(er) affinity, respectively. In other words, primed Th cells that provide cognate T help to B cells recognizing one format of the Ag can simultaneously serve as noncognate/bystander Th cells to B cells recognizing the very same antigen presented in another format. Because of the distinct type of Th assistance (i.e., cognate versus noncognate) they are receiving from the same Th cells, priming of B cells that recognize different constellations of the same Ag can cause distinct memory B cells to produce Abs that – although directed at the same Ag – will bind to their target with different affinity. More specifically, the same exact Ag can induce both high-affinity Abs (i.e., triggered by its 'cognate'/immunodominant format) and low-affinity Abs (i.e., triggered by its 'noncognate'/immune subdominant format). In order for the different antigenic formats to prime memory B cells while both receiving assistance from the same T helper cells, it is imperative that:

> i) the different formats of the same Ag are not (co-)localized to the same Ag carrier (e.g., free- circulating virus or free-circulating S protein released from mRNA-transfected cells), as this would otherwise allow the immunodominant antigenic format to outcompete the immune subdominant antigenic format

> ii) in one format, the T helper Ag and Bc Ag are co-localized to the same free circulating carrier (e.g., free-circulating

virus). As the latter will be taken up and processed by APCs, CD4+ T cells will be primed that provide cognate T help to the co-localized Bc antigen (and thereby enable priming of functional Abs of high affinity) while equally serving as bystander Th cells to assist priming of low-affinity Abs to the same Ag that is simultaneously expressed on a neighboring, non-circulating carrier (e.g., expressed at the surface of an mRNA-transfected cell). As the mRNA has been chemically altered to enhance its stability, it is highly likely that S protein is still expressed on the surface of mRNA-transfected cells by the time free-circulating S protein is internalized into APCs after having been released from mRNA-transfected cells into the peripheral tissue

iii) the non-circulating format of the target antigen (e.g., S protein in the case of Coronavirus [CoV]) binds with sufficient affinity to BCRs on naïve B cells to stimulate these cells

It is important to note that recall of SC-2-specific memory Th helper cells induced upon previous productive infection can equally provide noncognate T help to assist priming of low affinity anti-S memory B cells upon post-infection administration of a single mRNA vaccine dose.

From the above it can be concluded that cell surface-expressed viral target proteins synthesized by mRNA-transfected cells (i.e., S protein in case of SC-2) can rapidly recall previously primed memory B cells that produce anti-S Abs of low affinity, irrespective of whether priming of these B cells occurred as a result of a primary mRNA vaccine series or as a result of administration of a single mRNA dose following productive infection. S protein-associated epitopes that are expressed on the surface of host cells at an early stage of productive infection with SC-2 or *in vivo* S protein synthesis following mRNA vaccination (i.e., before the virus or S protein is released from SC-2-infected or mRNA-transfected host cells, respectively) can readily recall previously primed, S-specific memory B cells that – because of the noncognate T help they received – secrete Abs of low affinity[13].

In both instances, previously primed memory B cells of low affinity can be recalled by trimeric spike protein (or other homomultimeric viral proteins such as homotrimeric hemagglutinin [HA] in the case of Influenza virus, for example) that is expressed at the surface of the mRNA-transfected or virus-infected cell. Cell surface expression of S antigen in repetitive patterns results in recall of memory B cells producing Abs that bind with low affinity, not only to cell surface-expressed S protein[14] but also to free-circulating S protein Ag as soon as the latter is released from mRNA-transfected host cells, or to S protein expressed on the surface of progeny virus as soon as the latter is released from virus-infected host cells. These Abs will therefore circulate before cognate S-associated epitopes expressed on free-circulating virus or free circulating S protein released from virus-infected or mRNA-transfected host cells respectively, are presented by tissue-resident APCs to recall previously primed cognate Th-dependent anti-S Abs.

More specifically, mRNA boosting or productive infection following administration of a primary series of mRNA-based vaccine injections, or mRNA-based vaccine injections in previously infection-primed or vaccine-primed persons, will allow for recalled anti-S Abs to bind with low affinity to their respective immunodominant epitopes expressed on the surface of the free circulating S protein (in case of mRNA vaccination/boosting), or the free circulating SC-2 virions (in the case of infection) prior to uptake of S protein or SC-2 virus into tissue-resident APCs.

Recall of Abs that bind with low affinity to their respective epitopes expressed on virus surface-expressed or free-circulating S protein is thought to trigger SIR by masking S-associated immunodominant epitopes (fig. 3).

This prevents high-affinity (i.e., cognate Th-dependent) B cell immune responses to S protein from being recalled while enabling immune subdominant epitopes to take advantage of recalled S- or SC-2-specific CD4+ T cells (via internalization of free circulating S protein or free circulating virus into APCs) for providing noncognate T help to assist priming of low-affinity memory B cells directed at more conserved, immune subdominant epitopes. Noncognate Th-dependent priming of these memory B cells is thought to be responsible for inducing broadly cross-neutralizing Abs towards these more conserved, immune subdominant S-associated epitopes.

The observation that sera from triple mRNA-vaccinated individuals exhibited broadly neutralizing activity sharply contrasts with the results from neutralization assays performed on plasma from individuals who received a booster dose six months after two doses of an inactivated vaccine (ref. 26) or a non-replicating adenovector-based vaccine (ref. 29). Boosting with these vaccines resulted in a substantial drop of neutralizing capacity towards newly emerged Omicron sublineages. In the case of non-replicating viral vector vaccines, the S-encoding mRNA is directly transcribed from the DNA insert without exogenous chemical modification. It is therefore likely that the viral intracellular mRNA is degraded before the secreted, free-circulating S protein is presented to Ag-specific CD4+ T cells after uptake into APCs. This corroborates the above-proposed role of cell surface-expressed S protein in facilitating priming of low affinity anti-S Abs as mRNA-transfected but not adenovector-infected cells enable cell surface expression of S protein.

1.2.2. How can mRNA-based vaccines, but not natural infection, trigger immune refocusing?

Viruses – similar to some other pathogens - produce pathogen-derived self-mimicking peptides (PSMPs) most likely comprised within DRiPs (defective ribosomal products[15]) that are capable of silencing immune recognition at an early stage of viral infection by hijacking antigen presentation and thereby compromising the induction of CD4+ T helper cells (*G. Vanden Bossche, withdrawn provisional patent application*). mRNA vaccine technology, however, does not allow for production of PSMPs and hence does not prevent APCs from generating Th cells capable of assisting the priming of Bc responses towards foreign viral proteins that are expressed at the surface of the mRNA-transfected cells (i.e., prior to protein release from the transfected cell).

Based on all the above, it is reasonable to postulate that S-associated epitopes displayed on circulating S protein and multimeric patterns of S protein expressed on the surface of mRNA-transfected cells can take advantage of cognate and noncognate T help respectively to induce memory B cells that recognize S-specific Bc epitopes with high and low(er) affinity, respectively. It is also plausible that productive infection following a primary series of mRNA vaccinations or administration of an mRNA-based vaccine dose to previously infection- or vaccine-primed individuals[16] recalls anti-S Abs that bind with low affinity to S-associated immunodominant epitopes, regardless of whether the S protein involved is derived from the original Wuhan-Hu lineage or from a more recent Omicron descendant. New immune responses generated by mRNA-based booster vaccines, including the bivalent mRNA-based booster[17] dose and other potential Omicron-adapted mRNA-based booster shots, could at most induce low-affinity Abs that only provide short-lived protection regardless of whether they target more conserved, broadly neutralizing or infection-facilitating epitopes. Given the current co-circulation of highly infectious Omicron descendants, Omicron-adapted booster vaccines no longer enable immune refocusing and can no longer prime new Abs to either immunodominant or immune subdominant S-associated epitopes (chapters 1.2.10. and 7.2).

In conclusion, mRNA transfection of host cells following priming with vaccines or natural infection, or priming by a primary series of mRNA vaccinations followed by productive infection, are prone to suppress high-affinity anti-S immune responses to variable immunodominant S-associated Bc epitopes. Instead, all of these scenarios educate the immune system of the vaccinated individual to mount new, low-affinity anti-S Abs to more conserved, immune subdominant Bc epitopes. mRNA vaccination alone or in combination with productive infection promotes SIR.

1.2.3. PNNAb-dependent BTIs in vaccinated individuals are also a major driver of SIR and thus of viral immune escape.

Immune refocusing from immunodominant to immune subdominant S-associated epitopes not only occurs when low-affinity Abs are induced against homologous S protein on which the immunodominant epitopes have been masked, but can also be triggered when previously primed anti-S Abs bind with low affinity to S-associated epitopes expressed on a heterologous S protein variant. The latter typically occurs when pre-existing anti-S Abs are exposed to new emerging Omicron descendants which they can no longer sufficiently neutralize. Since the advent of Omicron, SIR has become a major driver of immune escape in highly vaccinated populations. But how does it work?

I postulate that binding of high concentrations of pre-existing, poorly neutralizing Abs to the S protein of dominantly circulating OOV triggered changes in viral colloidal behavior and promoted formation of weak viral aggregates. Viral aggregation would allow the highly conserved, immunocryptic site on the N-terminal domain of S protein (S-NTD) to present in multimeric arrays on the surface of these aggregates and thereby serve as a Th-independent Bc antigen. Triggering B cells with BCRs that recognize these repetitive antigenic patterns would lead to the production of polyreactive, non-neutralizing Abs (PNNAbs) that bind to the conserved antigenic site within S-NTD and thereby enhance viral infectiousness (refs. 2, 3, 4 and 5). Enhanced viral infectiousness triggers PNNAb-dependent BTIs and therefore causes a high production rate of progeny virus.

It is reasonable to postulate that this may prevent pNAbs from binding in sufficient concentration on S protein expressed on the surface of progeny virions to ensure rapid internalization into professional APCs (chapters 1.2.3. and 1.2.4.). Instead, weak-affinity binding of pre-existing pNAbs to the immunodominant, S-associated epitopes would now lead to steric masking of these epitopes (fig. 3). Such BTIs will therefore redirect the immune response away from the immunodominant epitopes towards a series of more conserved,

11

immune subdominant epitopes. This illustrates how SIR can be elicited by BTIs that occur in the presence of a high concentration of poorly neutralizing anti-S Abs. High titers of anti-S Abs are typically induced by vaccines and can explain why PNNAb-dependent VBTIs trigger SIR regardless of the type of vaccine used (figs. 5 and 7).

1.2.4. Despite vaccine-mediated immune imprinting, PNNAb-mediated VBTIs do not recall vaccinal Abs and therefore provoke a second round of SIR. Whereas SIR-1 refocuses the immune response towards conserved S-associated antigenic domains that are broadly susceptible to virus neutralization, SIR-2 re-orients the immune response towards conserved antigenic domains that broadly facilitate viral infectiousness.

In line with the concept of 'original antigenic sin' (also called 'immune imprinting'), PNNAb-dependent VBTIs recall previously vaccine-primed CD4+ Th cells. SIR 1-enabling VBTIs prevent recall of vaccinal Abs (i.e., specific to the ancestral Wuhan-Hu S protein) while enabling recalled CD4+ Th cells to assist *de novo* priming of broadly neutralizing Abs directed at more conserved, S-associated immune subdominant domains (fig. 3). As these Abs are short-lived and have low affinity, widespread VBTIs will rapidly lead to high population-level immune pressure on the subdominant antigenic regions (fig. 6 ❶) and thereby result in co-emergence and co-circulation of several new immune escape variants. The pre-existing vaccine- and SIR-primed pNAbs will fail to neutralize these new emerging variants but still bind to their respective S-associated epitopes. Once again, binding of these pre-existing pNAbs to their S-associated epitopes will trigger clustering of SC-2 virions into weak aggregates that present multimeric arrays of the highly conserved, S-NTD-associated antigenic determinant at their surface, thereby eliciting Th-independent PNNAbs. By binding to the conserved antigenic site within S-NTD, these Abs enhance viral infectiousness and cause these new emerging immune escape variants to readily provoke another round of PNNAb-dependent VBTIs. The latter trigger SIR 2 and thereby promote low-affinity binding between the mutated S protein on progeny virus and the pre-existing S-specific pNAbs (fig. 3).

Recall of previously vaccine-primed CD4+ Th cells combined with SIR 2 enables noncognate Th-dependent *de novo* priming of Abs that are redirected at more conserved, broadly infection-facilitating epitopes comprised within S-NTD.

To my knowledge, no data has been reported on the affinity maturation of these broadly conserved infection-inhibiting Abs. However, analogous to previously *de novo* primed broadly neutralizing Abs, their priming depends on noncognate T help. It is therefore reasonable to assume it may take several months for the corresponding memory B cells to undergo sufficient affinity maturation to ensure strong infection-inhibitory capacity in sera of convalescents who experienced such PNNAb-dependent VBTI. This would explain why protection against infection of vaccinated individuals who recovered from VBTIs (or who received an mRNA booster dose (chapter 1.2.1.)) has been short-lived; cross-functional Abs elicited as a result of PNNAb-dependent VBTIs would have given rise to a rapid increase in humoral immune pressure on the corresponding more conserved S-associated epitopes and thereby expedited large-scale viral immune escape in highly C-19-vaccinated populations (fig. 6 ❷❸).

1.2.5. Why do broadly neutralizing anti-S Abs elicited upon SIR-enabling VBTIs or mRNA booster doses have lower affinity than the originally elicited vaccine-induced NAbs?

Immune refocusing allows the host immune system to develop some new neutralizing capacity after multiple mutations in previously circulating pre-Omicron variants diminished the neutralizing capacity of vaccine-induced S-specific NAbs. Whereas the latter were directed at a broad and diversified spectrum of dominant, variant-specific epitopes that are primarily situated within S-RBD, *de novo* primed NAbs target a limited subset of more conserved epitopes and have relatively low affinity. This explains why cross-neutralizing Ab titers elicited shortly after SIR-enabling VBTIs or after mRNA booster immunizations in previously mRNA vaccine-primed individuals rapidly declined.

Priming of early vaccine-induced neutralizing Abs directed against highly variable S-associated immunodominant epitopes on pre-Omicron variants was assisted by cognate T help. Cognate Th-dependent priming of anti-S Abs promotes affinity maturation. Consequently, vaccinal Abs targeted at S-associated immunodominant epitopes (primarily situated within S-RBD) rapidly gained enhanced virus-neutralizing capability. In contrast, SIR-mediated priming of broadly neutralizing Abs elicited against more conserved, S-associated subdominant domains is assisted by CD4+ T memory cells which are recalled upon internalization of free-circulating virus (in the case of VBTI) or free-circulating S protein (in the case of mRNA-based vaccination) into APCs and subsequent presentation of virus- or S-derived antigenic Th peptides. Provision of noncognate T help by these bystander Th cells may explain why it takes several months after SIR-enabling VBTI or mRNA booster vaccination for the *de novo* primed memory B cells to mature in germinal centers (refs. 29-31) and produce broadly neutralizing Abs of high affinity and enhanced virus-neutralizing capacity. As it is only with a considerable delay that these Abs gain enhanced virus-neutralizing capacity, they promote the emergence of new immune escape variants before they have acquired optimal affinity. The same likely applies to the affinity maturation of infection-inhibiting Abs elicited upon a subsequent SIR-enabling VBTI (i.e. fig. 3 provoking SIR-2) or administration of updated mRNA booster doses.

THE INESCAPABLE IMMUNE ESCAPE PANDEMIC

1.2.6. Omicron's strategy to enhance viral immune escape in highly vaccinated populations.

It cannot be denied that mass vaccination drove resistance of pre-Omicron variants to the variable immunodominant epitopes within S protein and was responsible for the emergence of Omicron.

But why did Omicron come up with more than thirty amino acid mutations in its S protein?

This is unprecedented!

The evolutionary significance of the sudden, spectacular expansion of OOV in highly vaccinated populations was to make sure that SIR-mediating VBTIs could take place on a large-scale to ultimately cause the population to place high and widespread immune pressure on *more conserved, vitally important epitopes*. Population-level immune pressure on the more conserved, immune subdominant antigenic domains drove large-scale emergence of new variants that were resistant to broadly neutralizing Abs, and eventually incorporated a shared subset of infection-enhancing domains in their S-RBD to also escape from increasing population-level immune pressure exerted by broadly infection-inhibiting Abs (figs. 6 and 9).

SIR-mediating VBTIs have indeed been fueling large-scale viral immune escape that has materialized in the co-emergence and co-circulation of an evolving series of multiple new (sub)variants. Lineages that picked up a limited set of variant-specific, RBD-associated infection-enhancing mutations have subsequently acquired a level of intrinsic infectiousness that was high enough to cause Ab-independent VBTIs and thereby abolished population-level immune pressure exerted by re-focused, low-affinity Abs on common, infection-facilitating domains comprised within S-NTD (figs. 6 and 9 C).

It is therefore fair to conclude that PNNAb-dependent VBTIs allowed highly vaccinated populations to shift their immune response abruptly and collectively from variant S-specific high-affinity Abs to variant S-nonspecific low-affinity Abs, leading to a rapid increase in immune pressure on viral infectivity (fig. 6).

However, in order for SC-2 to be able to induce this spectacular change, it needed to incorporate a sufficient number of S-associated mutations[18] . This enabled OOV to dramatically diminish the neutralizing capacity of previously elicited variant S-specific Abs and enhance the susceptibility of vaccinated individuals to infection. In this way, Omicron S protein could trigger widespread stimulation of Th-independent PNAAbs and thereby facilitate PNNAb-dependent VBTIs, which are a *conditio sine qua non* for provoking SIR. By re-orienting the immune response of highly vaccinated populations to broadly shared (i.e., more conserved) and vitally important, immune subdominant S-associated domains, SIR-enabling VBTIs primed broadly neutralizing or infection-inhibiting low-affinity Abs that rapidly exerted large-scale immune pressure on these subdominant antigenic domains. Because highly vaccinated populations placed immune pressure on more conserved, vitally important S-associated antigenic domains, a diversified subgroup of circulating Omicron [sub]variants that had picked up the same limited subset(s) of variant-specific immune escape mutations could gain the same competitive advantage and start to co-circulate (fig. 9). This explains why and how OOV rapidly promoted co-circulation of new Omicron sub lineages that were resistant to OOV-induced humoral immunity, thereby dramatically expediting the evolutionary dynamics of immune escape.

Whereas PNNAb-*dependent* VBTIs caused new, broadly cross-reactive Abs generated in vaccinees to rapidly place high but short-lived immune pressure on *viral infectiousness*, co-circulation of newly emerged, highly infectious Omicron descendants eventually triggered PNNAb-*independent* VBTIs that caused highly vaccinated populations to place widespread, gradually increasing immune pressure on viral *trans infectiousness* (chapter 1.2.10.).

Although both PNNAb-dependent and PNNAb-independent VBTIs diminish viral shedding (chapters 3.2. and 3.3.), gradually increasing immune pressure on viral *trans infectiousness* is highly likely to drive selection of variants that combine NAb-evasiveness, enhanced infectiousness, and greater virulence in highly vaccinated populations (chapters 1.2.10. and 3.1.). Because mRNA-based vaccines promote SIR and because SIR expedites immune escape, it is reasonable to postulate that PNNAb-mediated immune pressure will rise more rapidly and drastically in populations that have been subject to mass vaccination with mRNA-based vaccines.

In summary, OOV and EOSVs have been responsible for a large wave of VBTIs in massively vaccinated countries. PNNAb-mediated VBTIs drive SIR, which subsequently fuels new VBTIs (figs. 4, 5 and 7). As mRNA vaccines also enable SIR, it is likely that mass vaccination with mRNA-based vaccines amplified and accelerated the wave of PNNAb-dependent VBTIs and hence, expedited co-emergence and co-circulation of pNAb-resistant Omicron-derived variants in highly vaccinated populations (figs. 1, 7 and 9).

More recently emerged Omicron descendants are, in addition, characterized by a high level of intrinsic infectiousness and are now putting vaccinees in highly vaccinated populations at risk of contracting AIESD (chapters 1.2.10. and 2.1.). It follows that mRNA-based booster injections and VBTIs have maximized NAb evasion in convalescent vaccinees and promoted resistance of new Omicron sublineages to Omicron-induced Abs (that will soon include PNNAbs).

1.2.7. PNNAb-dependent VBTIs enable highly vaccinated populations to rapidly re-orient cognate Th-dependent immune pressure on variable S-associated epitopes to noncognate Th-dependent immune pressure on more conserved S-associated epitopes. Subsequent Ab-independent VBTIs allow re-orientation of noncognate Th-dependent immune pressure on more conserved S-associated epitopes to Th-independent immune pressure on a highly conserved S-NTD-associated antigenic determinant. This evolution allows PNNAb-dependent or (PNN)Ab-independent VBTIs to cause fast and large-scale viral immune escape.

Whereas population-level immune pressure on viral infectiousness and neutralizability exerted by high-affinity S-specific vaccinal Abs gradually increased with progressive incorporation of more mutations of immunodominant epitopes in the variable S-RBD, population-level immune pressure on virus neutralizability and infectiousness exerted by broadly functional SIR-induced Abs rapidly grew due to delayed affinity maturation of *de novo* primed memory B cells.

High-affinity Abs with sub neutralizing activity towards *variable, immunodominant* S-associated epitopes drove sequential natural selection and dominant circulation of several more infectious and less neutralizable pre-Omicron immune escape variants. This trend continued until high population-level immune pressure on virus neutralizability in highly vaccinated populations led to natural selection and propagation of an immune escape variant (i.e., OOV) that sufficiently resisted vaccine-induced pNAbs to trigger large-scale VBTIs and thereby dramatically lowered population-level immune pressure on viral neutralizability (fig. 6 A). OOV enabled an abrupt shift from high to low humoral immune pressure on viral neutralizability through incorporation of an extensive arsenal of specific NAb-evasive mutations within S-RBD. This spectacular antigenic shift dramatically diminished the neutralizing capacity of Wuhan S-specific vaccinal Abs.

In contrast, low-affinity Abs with neutralizing activity towards *more conserved* (i.e., variant-nonspecific) *immune subdominant* S-associated epitopes drove co-emergence and co-circulation of several NAb-evasive Omicron-derived immune escape subvariants. This trend briefly continued until high population-level immune pressure on viral infectiousness in highly vaccinated populations led to co-emergence and co-circulation of highly infectious Omicron-derived immune escape variants capable of triggering Ab-independent VBTIs. The latter caused these populations to dramatically raise population-level immune pressure on viral *trans* infectiousness (fig. 6 C ❹).

The evolution of population-level immune pressure since the advent of Omicron is depicted in fig. 6. Below, I explain the immune mechanisms underlying the depicted immune pressure dynamics.

Following OOV-induced SIR 1-enabling VBTIs, immune escape from broadly neutralizing, low-affinity Abs occurred through convergent evolution of a limited subset of escape mutations that enriched the targeted, conserved S-NTD domain with epitopes more specific to the ancestral Wuhan-Hu lineage (refs. 30-32). This evolution rendered newly emerging Omicron descendants largely resistant to the pre-existing broadly neutralizing Abs. Following subsequent SIR 2-enabling VBTIs, immune escape from *de novo* induced broadly infection-inhibiting Abs with even lower affinity[19] occurred through incorporation of a limited subset of specific infection-enhancing mutations[20] that converged to the variable S-RBD (ref. 23). These converging mutations could still boost some previously vaccine-induced Abs and likely act in concert with one another to strengthen binding of SC-2 to human ACE2 (hACE2) such as to bolster intrinsic infectiousness of new emerging Omicron descendants. Consequently, more recently emerged Omicron-derived lineages are now combining pNAb-resistance with a *high level of viral infectiousness.*

By enriching conserved regions of their S-NTD or S-RBD with a limited but shared subset of specific NAb-evasive mutations or specific infection-enhancing mutations respectively, new emerging Omicron-derived variants drove *large-scale* immune escape. This explains the current *co-circulation* of a diverse subset[21] of highly infectious Omicron-derived sublineages (fig. 9). Because of their diversity and convergent evolution of additional (infection-enhancing) mutations to their S-RBD, the antigenic characteristics of co-circulating, highly infectious Omicron descendants have become more distant from those featuring the OOV. *Ab-independent VBTIs* triggered by any of the highly infectious, co-circulating Omicron descendants will contribute to enhancing PNNAb-mediated population-level immune pressure on the conserved antigenic site within S-NTD[22]. It is therefore fair to postulate that co-circulating highly infectious Omicron descendants experience the same population-level immune pressure on viral virulence. Any of these variants that acquire O-glycosite mutations allowing for enhanced intrinsic virulence will likely cause severe disease in a limited number of vaccinees.

I postulate that the current dominant expansion of XBB.1.5. illustrates a selection bias towards O-glycosite mutations that enable enhanced virulence without substantial fitness cost (chapter 3.4.1.). It seems likely that this variant is going to expand glycosylation of its S-associated O-glycosite mutation as a function of the increasing pace at which the population-level immune pressure on viral virulence is growing (ref. 5). As this pace is thought to grow exponentially in highly vaccinated populations, I predict that such a variant could soon unchain a surge of AIESD (figs. 6 and 9).

1.2.8. Rapid immune escape from refocused humoral immune responses elicited by VBTIs with Omicron relies on *convergent devolution* of a limited subset of more conserved S-NTD or S-RBD domains to antigenic determinants that are derived from the ancestral Wuhan-Hu lineage or pre-Omicron variants, respectively.

It is interesting to note how viral adaptation to suboptimal population-level immune pressure on conserved (i.e., variant-nonspecific) S-associated peptide epitopes has been driving natural selection of new immune escape variants that enriched their S-NTD and S-RBD region with antigenic determinants derived from the ancestral Wuhan-Hu lineage and specific successively dominating pre-Omicron variants respectively to evade broadly neutralizing or infection-inhibiting Abs in convalescent sera from vaccinated individuals.

Affinity maturation of broadly neutralizing Abs following mRNA booster shots in previously mRNA vaccine-primed people or or individuals who experienced VBTIs has been reported to be delayed (refs. 29, 30 and 31). This may explain why the protective effect of these NAbs has been short-lived. In addition, SIR-enabling VBTIs drive selective population-level immune pressure to promote *convergent devolution* (i.e., backward evolution) of more conserved NTD-associated sequences to antigenic determinants *that are specific to the Wuhan-Hu S Ag* (i.e., the S protein version of the ancestral lineage) [refs. 30, 31 and 32]. New emerging variants that have picked up a shared subset of these ancestral antigenic determinants managed to escape from these broadly neutralizing Abs and triggered new PNNAb-mediated VBTIs.

Subsequent binding of pre-existing affinity-matured pNAbs to their S-associated immunodominant and subdominant epitopes (i.e., primed by the vaccine and SIR 1, respectively) triggered an additional round of SIR (i.e. fig. 3 SIR 2). Along the same lines of reasoning, SIR 2 is thought to prime yet another set of anti-S Abs that bind with even lower affinity to more conserved, S-NTD-associated antigenic determinants and thereby exert rapidly increasing selective immune pressure on the infectiousness of all previously selected co-circulating Omicron-derived lineages. It is reasonable to assume that large-scale immune pressure on viral infectiousness drove natural selection of circulating Omicron descendants that separately incorporated a subset of the *same infection-enhancing antigenic determinants*[23] to reach a similarly high level of intrinsic viral infectiousness. As SIR drives *large-scale* immune escape, it is not surprising that this resulted in the co-emergence and co-circulation of Omicron descendants that convergently evolved their S-RBD by incorporating *variant S-specific* infection-enhancing determinants derived from previously dominantly circulating pre-Omicron variants (ref. 23). By provoking *Ab-independent* VBTIs, these highly infectious Omicron descendants will ultimately pave the way to unleashing viral virulence by causing vaccinated individuals to gradually augment PNNAb-mediated immune pressure on viral *trans* infectiousness (fig. 6 ❹). This is thought to drive natural selection of a more/highly infectious variant that has the appropriate O-glycosite mutation to enable high virulence in the majority of the vaccinated population (chapter 3.4.1.) (ref. 5).

Although I exclusively focused my analysis on mRNA-based vaccines, it is reasonable to assume that in the case of mass vaccination using other non-replicating vaccines (i.e., not based on mRNA technology), the very same convergent evolution of S-NTD and S-RBD occurred. However, the critically important difference is that administration of a primary series of vaccinations comprising a single mRNA-based vaccine shot is already sufficient to trigger SIR upon post-vaccination infection of previously infection-inexperienced individuals (fig. 1).

In summary, as the affinity of the S variant-specific NAbs matured, the RBD-constellation of SC-2 dramatically changed (i.e., Omicron) to facilitate PNNAb-enhanced viral infectiousness and thereby force the host immune system to focus its immune response on subdominant, more conserved S-associated domains (via SIR 1-enabling VBTIs). SIR 1 generated broadly neutralizing Abs of *low affinity* that rapidly[24] placed high immune pressure on viral neutralizability and thereby drove convergent evolution of ancestral virus-neutralizing motifs to S-NTD. This prompted rapid and large-scale immune escape from broadly NAbs. The resulting immune escape variants triggered SIR 2-enabling VBTIs that rapidly led to convergent evolution of variant-specific infection-enhancing motifs to S-RBD and thereby gave rise to co-emergence and co-circulation of *highly infectious* Omicron descendants. The latter are now triggering Ab-independent VBTIs that cause highly vaccinated populations to gradually raise PNNAb-mediated immune pressure on viral *trans* infectiousness/virulence (fig. 6 ❹).

1.2.9. To maximize the effect on viral immune escape, SIR-1–following VBTIs with OOV–had to precede SIR-2.

Subsequent to OOV-mediated VBTI, SIR occurred in 2 different stages: SIR 1 and SIR 2.

To maximize viral immune escape, SIR had to occur in two different stages whereby large-scale immune pressure on broadly neutralizing, low-affinity Abs was followed by large-scale immune pressure on broadly infection-inhibiting Abs that presumably had even lower affinity,[25] and thus provided an even shorter duration of protection from productive infection. Clinical data on sera from convalescent or mRNA-boosted vaccinated individuals[26] seem to indicate that a SIR-2-enabling event was preceded by a SIR-1-enabling event. I postulate that in order for a VBTI to efficiently foster viral immune escape, this must be the case.

Successive occurrence of both SIR-1 and SIR-2 ensures that SIR-2 occurs at a time when previously primed broadly neutralizing Abs have sufficiently matured to allow their binding to new emerging Omicron-derived immune escape [sub]variants. Binding of pre-existing affinity-matured Abs in low but sufficient concentration to immunodominant S-associated epitopes on new pNAb-evasive lineages seems critical to enable SIR-1. However, SIR-1-induced NAbs are directed at multiple subdominant S-associated epitopes. Avidity maturation of the corresponding S-specific memory B cells is therefore likely to enable binding of multiple sub neutralizing Abs to S protein. This would (normally?) be expected to promote virus uptake into APCs and hamper SIR. However, avidity maturation of Abs directed at S-associated subdominant epitopes is thought to cause a relative increase in S-reactive, IgG4 switched B cells. As IgG4 Abs have reduced Fc-mediated effector function (ref. 29), they likely delay virus uptake into APCs. Virus-pNAb complexes would therefore be more likely to trigger SIR-2. Delayed maturation resulting in increased levels of IgG4 Abs has been reported to occur after the second vaccination with mRNA-based vaccines. As an mRNA booster dose elicited a broadly neutralizing Ab response (ref. 29), it is reasonable to assume that the increase in IgG4 Abs was caused by the induction of low-affinity Abs towards the immune subdominant format of S protein expressed at the surface of mRNA-transfected cells. As previously explained, mRNA-based vaccines are thought to promote SIR due to their capacity to elicit such low-affinity Abs (see chapters 1.2.1. and 1.2.2.).

Despite a temporary decline in viral transmission rates in highly vaccinated populations (presumably due to broadly neutralizing or infection-inhibiting activity of refocused Ab responses in convalescent and mRNA-boosted vaccinees), SIR (i.e., SIR-1 and SIR-2 combined) enabled a spectacular shift and increase in humoral immune pressure on the infectiousness of previously co-circulating Omicron [sub]variants (fig. 6 ❷❸). The above evolution explains how and why dominant circulation of OOV rapidly paved the way for co-circulation of a diversified subgroup of highly infectious Omicron descendants (fig. 9).

GEERT VANDEN BOSSCHE, DVM, PHD

1.2.10. Once highly infectious Omicron descendants circulate, neither additional vaccination (e.g., additional booster doses or vaccination of additional age groups such as children) nor a complete halt of the mass vaccination program will be able to prevent highly vaccinated populations from increasing immune pressure on viral virulence.

Halting the mass vaccination experiment or, on the contrary, further expanding it no longer has any influence on the likelihood for new, more virulent variants to emerge. Whereas previous Omicron descendants were self-catalyzing large-scale immune escape in highly vaccinated populations as a result of SIR-enabling VBTIs, more recently emerged Omicron descendants have high intrinsic infectiousness and trigger VBTIs in a way that is fully Ab-independent. This is because highly infectious Omicron descendants cause productive infection before pre-existing vaccine-induced pNAbs have a chance to bind. Consequently, they do not stimulate PNNAbs prior to their hACE2-mediated entry into susceptible epithelial cells. While SIR-enabling VBTIs are triggered by PNNAbs, highly infectious Omicron [sub]variants no longer trigger SIR and therefore no new cross-functional Abs can be elicited following VBTIs with these new variants. On the contrary, exposure to highly infectious variants will promote attachment of SC-2 progeny virions to the surface of migratory DCs (ref. 40) and thereby diminish the concentration of PNNAbs adsorbed to DC-tethered SC-2 virions. In this way, widespread (re-)exposure of a highly vaccinated population raises PNNAb-mediated population-level immune pressure on viral virulence (see chapter 1.2.4.).

In addition, vaccines (i.e., updated, Omicron-adapted booster doses) will be unable to prevent recurrent Ab-independent VBTIs in vaccinated individuals from driving a gradual increase in population-level immune pressure on viral *trans* infectiousness/virulence. This is because additional booster doses can at most recall previously vaccine-primed pNAbs; they can no longer prime new functional S-specific Abs, regardless of the antigenic characteristics of the Omicron-adapted S protein in the vaccine. Failure to prime new NAbs is due to the fact that re-exposure to highly infectious variants causes a steadily growing concentration of free progeny virions (i.e., exceeding the maximal rate of viral adsorption by migratory DCs) that are captured by the pre-existing vaccinal Abs and thereby outcompete the vaccinal Ag for uptake and presentation by professional Ag-presenting cells (fig. 11) (chapters 8.2. and 11.9.).

Based on the above, it is reasonable to conclude that PNNAb-mediated VBTIs triggered SIR-1 and SIR-2, and that the ensuing emergence of new immune escape variants allowed broadly virus-neutralizing or broadly infection-inhibiting Abs to exert a high level of large-scale immune pressure on more conserved S-NTD-associated epitopes. Such high and large-scale immune pressure rapidly led to co-circulation of a diversified subset of highly infectious variants that are largely resistant to vaccine-induced pNAbs and cannot prime *de novo* immune responses. These new emerging variants provoke Ab-independent VBTIs that cause highly infectious viral virions to dilute the concentration of PNNAbs adsorbed on the surface of URT-resident DCs and thereby place gradually increasing PNNAb-mediated immune pressure on viral virulence (fig. 11). Booster doses with the original, Wuhan-Hu-based vaccine could at most boost vaccinal pNAbs and thereby prolong production of PNNAbs upon restimulation following viral exposure. At best, this will delay, but not halt, the ongoing increase in PNNAb-mediated immune pressure on viral virulence. The same applies to extending vaccine coverage to unvaccinated segments of the population (e.g., children). This may temporarily dilute PNNAb-mediated population-level immune pressure, but will not prevent it from growing even more rapidly thereafter (due to more individuals exerting immune pressure on the virus).

I cannot imagine that anyone able to comprehend the adaptive evolutionary dynamics of SC-2 in the face of the evolving population-level immune pressure (as summarized in figs. 4, 6 and 9) would deny that highly vaccinated populations are heading towards an unprecedented public health calamity. Nor can I imagine a belief that additional vaccination will diminish the imminent threat from newly emerging more virulent variants that will inevitably put highly vaccinated countries at risk of a massive wave of AIESD.

1.2.11. It is impossible to understand the disastrous evolution of this immune escape pandemic without understanding SIR, i.e., without an understanding of how Omicron and mRNA-based vaccinations reshaped the affinity and breadth of the humoral anti-S response in vaccinated individuals.

On one hand, all mutation trackers seem concerned about additional S-associated mutations that endow newly emerging Omicron variants with a high level of intrinsic viral infectiousness, thereby rendering them resistant to both the vaccinal Abs and broadl+y neutralizing or infection-inhibiting *de novo* Abs elicited after previous mRNA booster doses or PNNAb-mediated VBTIs. On the other hand, researchers have not been serious about addressing the health risk associated with the emergence of such highly infectious Omicron (sub)variants other than proposing intensified surveillance. I can only conclude *they do not realize that,* since the advent of Omicron, SIR-enabling VBTIs and vaccinations (i.e., mRNA-based vaccination) have increasingly shifted effector mechanisms involved in vaccine-mediated protection from *high-affinity* humoral responses directed at *variable* S-associated epitopes (i.e., mediated by variant S-specific, *cognate T help-dependent* NAbs), to *low-affinity* humoral responses directed at *more conserved* S-associated epitopes (i.e., consecutively mediated by *noncognate Th-dependent* broadly infection-neutralizing Abs and *Th-independent* broadly virulence-neutralizing PNNAbs).

Low affinity anti-S Abs are prone to rapidly exert high immune pressure on viral reproduction and expedite viral immune escape. If low-affinity anti-S Abs are broadly cross-reactive, they will expedite *large-scale* immune escape. This applies particularly to Th-independent PNNAbs–these Abs are optimally suited for placing high and large-scale immune pressure on viral *trans* infectiousness/virulence.

Chapter Two

Ignoring Darwin's Theory

2.1. Mass vaccination during this pandemic has not contributed to building herd immunity but rather to building *herd* (i.e., population-level) *immune pressure* on SC-2 reproduction, and therefore prevented highly vaccinated countries from controlling viral transmission. Enhanced 'herd immune pressure' on Wuhan-Hu-specific S protein eventually led to natural selection of a spectacular and unique variant (i.e., OOV) that readily managed to dramatically diminish the neutralizing capacity of vaccine-induced pNAbs. The resulting SIR-enabling VBTIs have now led to co-selection and circulation of several highly infectious [sub]variants that fully evade pNAbs elicited by vaccines and provoke new VBTIs that fuel immune escape from virulence-inhibiting Abs (i.e., PNNAbs).

There is only one natural force behind the complex evolutionary dynamics of SC-2 that have been shaping the course of this pandemic in ways that are unprecedented. Regardless of mankind's interventions, this natural force is laid down in one of the key ideas of Darwin's theory:

Variants/mutants that, in a hostile environment, have a competitive advantage will be naturally selected to reproduce and dominate. Regardless of the stage of their adaptive evolution, growing pressure on the ability of an infectious organism to replicate and transmit will result in natural selection and expansion of mutants that exhibit a higher level of 'fitness', which for viruses translates into enhanced viral infectiousness.

While the virus adapts to large-scale humoral immune pressure exerted by highly vaccinated populations, vaccinated individuals mature their adaptive immune response. However, natural immune adaptation to SC-2 virus (and other viruses causing acute self-limiting infection) also includes epigenetic adaptation of the CBIIS (involving functional reprogramming of self-centered innate immune effector cells). This particularly applies to situations where the susceptible host is repeatedly exposed to changed (e.g., 'more infectious') environmental conditions (refs. 52 and 53). C-19 vaccines do not contain a replicating virus and therefore only induce an adaptive immune response. The latter is, however, insufficient for vaccinated individuals to successfully deal with SC-2 (and other viruses causing acute self-limiting infection) when they are exposed to the virus while their vaccinal Abs have not yet fully matured. This is typically the case when vaccination campaigns are started during a viral pandemic.

Although enhanced maturation of vaccine-induced Abs eventually acquired optimal neutralizing capacity towards the originally circulating lineage (i.e., Wuhan-Hu), their affinity-maturation did not lead to diminished population-level immune pressure on viral infectivity (i.e., infection rates in highly vaccinated populations did not decline). This is because another more infectious variant had already been selected and dominantly circulated by the time vaccine-induced, S variant-specific Abs had reached full-fledged maturity. As affinity-matured Abs are highly specific, their neutralizing capacity towards new SC-variants that had evolved additional mutations of one or more S-RBD-associated neutralizing epitopes (along with those that enhanced intrinsic infectiousness) became even worse. This eventually increased 'herd' immune pressure on the virus to a level sufficient to promote selection and dominant propagation of OOV.

OOV made the situation much worse by triggering widespread VBTIs in highly vaccinated populations. As previously mentioned, VBTIs led to 2 episodes of rapid but short-lived declines in herd/population-level immune pressure (i.e., via SIR-1 and SIR-2) that were then followed by a corresponding increase: steep (after SIR-1, SIR-2 and co-emergence of highly infectious Omicron descendants), or more gradual (after inflection point C) [fig. 6].

High and large-scale population-level immune pressure on viral infectiousness likely enabled the currently observed co-circulation of highly infectious Omicron descendants. These descendants contribute to generating large-scale and increasing immune pressure on viral virulence in highly vaccinated populations. This provides ample opportunity for SC-2 to generate and select new variants capable of evolving adequate O-glycosite mutations that enable them to escape from the increasing population-level immune pressure, even beyond a threshold sufficient to cause AIESD (chapters 3.4., 3.4.1. and 4.2.).

2.2. Viruses (causing acute self-limiting infections) will always stay ahead of life-threatening immune pressure exerted on the virus by adaptive host immunity.

To counter the effect of NAb affinity maturation during the pre-Omicron stage of this pandemic, the virus had to evolve an immune escape strategy that forced the immune system to reorient its NAb response to *low-affinity* Abs in order to rapidly augment population-level immune pressure on viral infectivity after a short-lived episode of immune protection. This could only be achieved if the virus changed its S-RBD in such a way to dramatically diminish the virus-neutralizing capacity of vaccine-induced pNAbs.

By incorporating over thirty single point mutations, fifteen of which occurred in the S-RBD (ref. 6), Omicron has been able to sufficiently diminish the neutralizing capacity of vaccinal Abs and hence triggered PNNAb-mediated VBTIs instead of further boosting pre-existing vaccinal pNAbs (as pre-Omicron variants previously did according to the concept of 'original antigenic sin'). PNNAb-dependent VBTIs ensured an enhanced productive infection rate in vaccinated individuals who previously experienced SIR and therefore possessed an inadequately trained CBIIS (fig. 5 panel C). Because of the high concentration of progeny virus in vaccinated individuals, pre-existing pNAbs could only bind in relatively low concentration to the virus and thereby triggered steric masking of S-associated immunodominant epitopes. This prompted priming of new, low-affinity Abs to more conserved, immune subdominant epitopes of S protein.

Consequently, selection and dominant propagation of Omicron has not been a mere coincidence but resulted solely from a logical evolutionary constraint imposed by raising 'herd' immune pressure placed on virus neutralizability as a result of the increasing percentage of vaccinated individuals developing high titers of high-affinity anti-S Abs (fig. 6 ❶). The spectacular loss of NAb capacity brought about by OOV rendered vaccinated individuals more susceptible to infection (via PNNAb-mediated *enhancement of viral infectiousness* (figs. 2, 4 and 8)) and thereby fulfilled the requirement for triggering widespread PNNAb-mediated VBTIs in highly vaccinated populations. These VBTIs shifted the humoral immune response from high titers of variant S-specific pNAbs of high affinity to relatively low titers of broadly functional S-specific Abs of low affinity.

Based on the above, one can understand how the advent of Omicron ignited a fulminant acceleration of evolutionary dynamics and expanded the spectrum of Omicron-derived subvariants. By enabling maximal immune escape, Omicron has ascertained optimal conditions for viral survival, including protection of vaccinated individuals from severe disease (via *PNNAb-mediate*d inhibition of severe disease (fig 10)).

In summary, evolutionary changes allowed the virus to rapidly adapt to population-level immune pressure on S-associated epitopes, irrespective of the type of targeted epitopes (i.e., dominant or subdominant) and the type of vaccine that led the population to exert that immune pressure. Vaccination with mRNA-based vaccines only expedited this evolution because of the low threshold necessary for mRNA-based vaccines to trigger SIR (fig. 1)

Those who pretend that intensified and expanded mass vaccination will allow the immune system of vaccinated individuals 'to stay ahead of the virus' do not grasp even the most basic tenets of evolutionary biology. This discipline unequivocally teaches that exactly the opposite applies!

Chapter Three

Omicron is now threatening to move from Ab-dependent enhancement of viral infectiousness to Ab-independent enhancement of viral virulence.

3.1. Why will the newly emerging, highly infectious Omicron-derived variants evolve towards enhanced virulence, and why will it take more time to reach this alarming outcome than previous mutational inflection points? (fig. 6 A, B, C, D)

Pre-existing anti-S Abs with strongly diminished neutralizing capability bind to the S-associated immunodominant epitopes of early Omicron lineages. As already mentioned, binding of pre-existing pNAbs to their S-associated immunodominant epitopes is postulated to promote viral aggregation. This enables the conserved enhancing site within S-NTD to establish a multimeric pattern on the surface of these (weak) viral aggregates and thereby elicits Th-independent[27] PNNAbs that bind with low affinity to S-NTD. Binding of PNNAbs to the conserved antigenic site within S-NTD is likely to trigger PNNAb-mediated VBTIs and inhibit *trans* infection,[28] preventing *trans* fusion of permissive cells in distal organs (including the lower respiratory tract; LRT)--a mechanism known to inhibit viral virulence (refs. 5 and 40-42). This also explains why vaccinated individuals no longer benefiting from short-lived, SIR-mediated protection from productive infection were still protected against severe disease (fig. 10).

Productive infection resulting from Ab-independent VBTIs with new Omicron-derived immune escape variants that separately incorporated a subset of shared infection-enhancing mutations to provide high intrinsic infectiousness results in a higher production rate of progeny virus and therefore more inflammation. This is thought to trigger adsorption of progeny virions onto the surface of migratory DCs patrolling the upper respiratory tract (URT) (ref. 40). There is *in vitro* evidence that binding of these DC-tethered virions by PNNAbs is responsible for preventing *trans* fusion and fusogenicity (formation of syncytia), which are generally acknowledged as pathognomonic for severe disease (refs. 40, 49, 50 and 56).

It is reasonable to postulate that following Ab-*independent* VBTI enhanced adsorption of progeny virions onto the surface of migratory DCs results in a reduced concentration of free progeny virions. Each free 'highly infectious' virion that is released from infected epithelial cells at the URT will therefore bind a relatively *higher* concentration of pre-existing pNAbs as compared to 'less infectious' progeny virions produced as a result of PNNAb-*dependent* VBTI. Abundant binding of pre-existing pNAbs to free progeny virions would no longer enable SIR (as in the case of PNNAb-dependent VBTIs) but promote weak aggregation of *progeny virus*. These weak viral aggregates would enable multimeric presentation of S-NTD and thereby stimulate production of PNNAbs while promoting abundant uptake of pNAb-complexed viral assemblies into APCs.

Enhanced viral uptake into APCs promotes elimination of virus-infected cells by MHC class I-unrestricted CTLs (i.e., presumably NK-CTLs) and therefore reduces viral shedding while promoting recovery from symptomatic VBTI[29] (ref. 43) (figs. 10-11). However, abundant uptake of SC-2 into APCs will also suppress presentation of other Ags, therefore suppressing the priming or recall of CD4+ T helper cells–helper cells that in turn assist priming or recall of immune effector B and T cells directed at other pathogenic agents (ref. 15) (chapter 11.9.).

As Th-independent PNNAbs are short-lived and have low affinity, their binding onto DC-tethered virions causes suboptimal population-level immune pressure on viral virulence and would normally only provide short-term protection against severe disease (fig. 10). However, once PNNAb-dependent VBTIs are replaced by PNNAb-independent VBTIs (i.e., upon co-circulation of highly infectious Omicron descendants), exposure to highly infectious variants likely results in a relatively higher rate of adsorption of progeny virions onto the surface of migratory DCs. Normally, this would rapidly increase PNNAb-mediated immune pressure on viral virulence. However, the increase in PNNAb-mediated immune pressure is likely mitigated by the enhanced production of PNNAbs following Ab-independent VBTIs (see above). This is likely to lead to a *gradual* rise in PNNAb-mediated population-level immune pressure on viral *trans* infectiousness/viral virulence in highly vaccinated populations, thereby providing adequate time for the virus to generate appropriate O-glycosite mutations that render new variants more virulent. Selection of more virulent variants will gradually improve the capacity of SC-2 to escape from the increasing selective immune pressure on viral virulence.

3.2. Enhanced protection of vaccinated individuals against disease is anything but a favorable prognostic sign.

As explained above, productive infection by highly infectious immune escape variants results in a high production rate of progeny virus. As long as vaccine-induced PNNAb titers are high enough, the enhanced viral production rate will cause diminished viral shedding and enhanced mitigation of disease symptoms via increased uptake of free SC-2 virions into tissue-resident DCs/APCs that facilitate CTL-mediated elimination of virus-infected cells.

Re-exposure to co-circulating highly infectious variants is therefore – for the time being – not only protecting vaccinated individuals against *severe* disease but against disease altogether (fig. 11). However, the steady diminishment in viral shedding and disease symptoms is inextricably linked to a steadily increasing population-level immune pressure on viral virulence.

It should therefore be acknowledged that the current expansion of co-circulating, highly infectious Omicron descendants is now causing highly vaccinated populations to increase PNNAb-mediated immune pressure on viral virulence. In other words, diminished viral shedding and improved protection against disease in vaccinated individuals have now become bad prognostic signs as they are inevitably associated with enhanced PNNAb-mediated immune pressure on viral *trans* infectiousness/virulence.

3.3. Why has Nature chosen to have highly vaccinated populations place suboptimal immune pressure on viral virulence rather than on viral shedding?

As MHC class I-unrestricted T cells are highly efficient in killing the virus (i.e., virus-infected cells), there is no immune pressure placed on viral shedding–no variants capable of evading this cytolytic immune function will be selected. In other words, highly vaccinated populations exposed to highly infectious Omicron descendants cannot exert cell-mediated immune pressure on the conserved, universal CTL peptide that is responsible for activation of said MHC class I-unrestricted T cells (refs. 5, 43 and 44). This universal peptide is not only targeted by NK-CTLs enabling elimination of productively infected host cells, but also by NK cells that – at an early stage of viral infection (i.e., before production of viral progeny takes place) – are capable of killing host cells infected with viruses causing acute self-limiting infections (G. Vanden Bossche, personal communication/unpublished research data).

Natural selection and widespread propagation of variants harboring a mutated universal CTL peptide would be catastrophic as it would prevent the immune system from controlling viral infection, regardless of the stage of infection. Such a mutation would allow SC-2 to universally[30] kill its host population during a pandemic, irrespective of the population's immune status (i.e., whether immunologically naïve or imprinted with innate cell-based or adaptive humoral memory). In other words, this MHC class I-unrestricted peptide is of vital importance to SC-2 and other CoVs–it is the key to restricting CoVs to acute, _self-limiting_ infections (and, for that matter, determining the self-limiting nature of pandemics themselves). Consequently, if the virus is to survive, it must pair diminished shedding (i.e., via augmented cytolytic killing of virus-infected cells or, for that matter, increased uptake of pNAb-complexed virions into APCs) with population-level immune pressure on another viral characteristic that is susceptible to natural selection and can compensate for diminished viral shedding.

As previously explained, reduced viral shedding is linked with increasing population-level immune pressure on viral *trans* infectiousness/virulence (as controlled by adsorption of PNNAbs onto DC-tethered virions) because both are inextricably triggered by a high level of intrinsic viral infectiousness. This explains why and how enhanced protection of vaccinated individuals against disease currently translates into progressively increasing PNNAb-mediated immune pressure on viral virulence in highly vaccinated populations.

3.4. Shifting to enhanced virulence has now become a matter of ensuring survival for the virus. How would the emergence of a highly virulent variant affect highly vaccinated countries and the evolution of the pandemic?

As recurrent Ab-independent VBTIs likely entail enhanced reduction of viral shedding (chapters 3.2 and 3.3.), the virus will eventually need to perform a spectacular rescue operation to safeguard its survival. As highly vaccinated populations are now collectively threatening SC-2 with diminished transmission[31] down to a level that becomes rate-limiting for viral survival, the S protein of the virus will need to shift towards a format that enables SC-2 to resist the inhibitory effect of variant S-nonspecific PNAAbs on viral *trans* infectiousness/virulence.

Since changes in the glycosylation profile of virus surface-expressed proteins may enable enhanced viral virulence and therefore be SC-2's last resort to ensure continued viral replication, I previously postulated that variants with a more extensive S-associated O-glycosylation profile would be selected to lift the blockade on viral virulence/*trans* infectiousness (ref. 5).

Before highly infectious variants started to circulate, the virus expedited its large-scale immune escape by forcing the immune system of vaccinated individuals to exert immune pressure on distinct, *more conserved* S-associated domains. SIR-enabling PNNAb-dependent VBTIs enabled *de novo* primed low-affinity Abs to broaden and expedite immune escape. By provoking Ab-independent VBTIs, highly infectious Omicron descendants have now managed to place increasing immune pressure on an *even more conserved* antigenic site comprised within S-NTD (ref. 5).

However, as viral shedding by vaccinated individuals is substantially diminishing, the virus has to choose a new approach to ensure its survival. Ideally, that approach would have to unleash viral virulence in a substantial part of the population.

However, as a fast and drastic reduction of the population size would not allow the virus to survive, enhanced viral virulence should (ideally) avoid a rapid decimation of the population. The smaller the part of the population affected by a highly virulent lineage and the slower the case fatality rate grows, the higher the likelihood the population can be sufficiently and timely replenished to control[32] the virus via herd immunity (instead of driving it into extinction for lack of sufficient viral transmission).

However, in the case of a massively vaccinated population, population-level immune pressure may eventually increase to a very high level (fig. 6 see curves in yellow). When the immune pressure exceeds a threshold sufficient to unleash a highly virulent variant (i.e., presumably endowed with a highly glycosylated O-glycosite mutation), a sudden and steep incline of mortality rates will ensue. This will prevent the population from building sufficient herd immunity.

Accelerated high mortality rates are a substitute for herd immunity in terms of their capacity to diminish transmission, but they do not ensure viral survival. Furthermore, due to continued exposure during the pandemic, only few (unvaccinated) individuals in highly vaccinated countries will have an inadequately trained CBIIS, and those who do will not serve as asymptomatic transmitters of the virus. Taken together, it is highly likely that huge waves of Ab-independent enhancement of severe disease will rapidly be followed by eradication of the highly virulent immune escape variant. This would terminate the immune escape pandemic. For the purpose of this manuscript, I am calling immune escape variants endowed with such highly glycosylated S-associated O-glycosite mutations 'HIVICRON', which stands for **hi**ghly **vi**rulent Omi**cron**-derived variants. HIVICRON is to be considered the common name for new Omicron-derived variants that are characterized by resistance to pNAbs and a level of intrinsic virulence that is high enough to cause widespread AIESD in highly vaccinated populations (chapter 3.4.1.)

3.4.1. How will the virus proceed with O-glycosylation of S protein to transition to a more virulent format?

By provoking Ab-independent VBTIs, the virus causes the immune system of a vaccinee to passively release the "immunological brakes," on viral *trans* infectiousness. Therefore unlike the case of SIR-mediated immune escape, there is no need for the virus to trigger VBTIs to prime new Ab responses that could subsequently exert immune pressure on viral reproduction.

It has not yet been described how immune-evasive O-glycosite mutations are selected. My understanding of their immune selection is as follows:

First, enhanced viral infectiousness leads to an enhanced viral production rate and therefore to a higher concentration of progeny virus. This implies that more progeny virions may be adorned with an S variant protein that happens to have an aberrant O-linked glycosylation profile. It is well known that numerous O-linked glycans can be produced by virus-infected cells as viral proteins pass through the Golgi apparatus. Moreover, it is likely that shifts in the distribution of distinct O-linked glycans occur, not only depending on amino acid mutations in viral glycoproteins but also on post-translational changes during processing of these viral glycoproteins in virus-infected cells (e.g., causing alterations to N-glycosylation) (refs. 7, 8).

It is currently not known whether enhanced intrinsic infectiousness of SC-2 could promote generation of other O-linked glycan cores (i.e., other than core-1 type O-glycans; ref. 9) that could subsequently be extended and processed to give rise to a more (diversified) O-glycosylation profile of S protein. However, this is likely to be the case as more infectious variants have already been reported to exhibit enhanced virulence *in vitro* (refs. 48-51 and 57). How N- and O-glycosylation of viral proteins, and S protein in particular, could subvert the host immune system and PNNAb-mediated inhibition of virulence in particular has been previously explained (ref. 5).

However, it is only when the immune pressure on PNNAb-mediated inhibition of viral *trans* infectiousness will collectively increase that large-scale selection of a unique S-associated, highly virulent PNNAb-evasive O-glycoform[33] (HIVICRON) could occur (fig. 6 and 9 D).

Increasing population-level immune pressure above a threshold sufficient to unleash a highly virulent SC-variant is more efficient if the immune pressure is exerted on a single variant instead of multiple co-circulating variants. This is why I assume O-glycosite mutations are currently driving selection and dominant propagation of a single Omicron descendant. My assumption is based on the following observations and reflections:

XBB lineages that resulted from recombination of distinct highly infectious BA.2-derived sub lineages have been reported to pair enhanced virulence (*in vitro*) with diminished intrinsic infectiousness (refs. 48 and 57). If enhanced virulence is due to O-glycosite mutations as previously postulated (ref. 5), diminished viral infectiousness could be explained by steric hindrance of host-cell entry by enhanced (O-)glycosylation of S-RBD. If O-glycosylation hampers viral entry, a specific S-associated O-glycosylation profile may be required in order for a new immune escape variant to become more virulent without further compromising its intrinsic infectiousness. A new emerging variant (e.g., derived from XBB or BQ.1) that incorporates such an adequate O-glycosite mutation would acquire a fitness advantage and therefore be selected to dominantly propagate. This may be the case for XBB.1.5, which now seems to increasingly supplant other co-circulating variants in highly vaccinated countries. Selection of a specific type of O-glycosite mutation is likely to lead to sequential dominant expansion in prevalence of more virulent variants (see solid yellow line in fig. 6 and dashed red line in fig. 9).

It is reasonable to assume that differential population-level immune pressure on viral virulence will select viral variants with differential levels of intrinsic virulence (fig. 6).

In countries/regions with lower vaccine coverage rates and limited use of mRNA-based vaccines, the level of immune pressure on viral virulence exerted by the population may not suffice to trigger transition of the dominantly circulating XBB.1.5. lineage into a highly virulent variant. In other words, additional glycosylation of S-associated O-glycosite mutations may not suffice to allow XBB.1.5. to breach the immune pressure mounted by the population and cause a steep increase in mortality rates. Countries/regions with lower vaccine coverage rates may therefore experience a protracted course of severe disease cases with more hospitalizations but fewer deaths. Such countries/regions may witness a high(er) incidence of chronic debilitating disease due to long-haul Covid.

On the other hand, in countries/regions with high vaccine coverage rates, especially if achieved through mRNA-based vaccination, population-level immune pressure may eventually reach a level high enough to trigger selection of an XBB.1.5.-derived variant that is equipped with a highly glycosylated O-glycosite mutation. The level of virulence of such a variant (i.e., HIVICRON) would be high enough to suddenly cause a massive surge of AIESD and thereby abolish the immune pressure on viral virulence exerted by the population.

Highly virulent variants will not spread widely; it is likely that—depending on the time required for the population-level immune pressure to exceed the threshold sufficient to unleash HIVICRON–waves of AIESD will unfold independently and at different timepoints in highly vaccinated countries.

A swift and steep decrease of population-level immune pressure on viral virulence *in vivo* (fig. 6 D) would entail a rapid and substantial decimation of highly vaccinated populations. Such a reduction in population size would greatly diminish viral transmission (depending on the case fatality rate), and given the vast majority of the remaining population (i.e., primarily, but not exclusively the unvaccinated) will have developed strong immune sterilizing capacity, the virus is likely to become eradicated (see above).

In summary, before high enough population-level immune pressure selects HIVICRON, XBB.1.5. may evolve distinct 'more virulent' S-associated O-glycoforms that weaken protection against severe disease in a growing subset of vaccinated individuals whose PNNAb titers have begun to fall below the optimal threshold for *in vivo* virulence-neutralizing capacity. This likely explains the currently observed upward trend in hospitalizations in several highly vaccinated countries.

As long as PNNAb titers have not collectively declined below this optimal threshold, the highly virulent O-glycosite mutant (HIVICRON) will not be selected and the virus will not yet *massively* break through the *in vivo* virulence-neutralizing capacity of vaccinatedindividuals.

However, when vaccinal titers start to decline in the majority of the vaccinated population, the conditions for generating high population-level immune pressure on viral virulence may be fulfilled. As this is expected to trigger the selection of HIVICRON, massive unlocking of viral virulence in vaccinated individuals will likely occur and provoke an explosion of cases of AIESD[34].

Based on the above, it can be argued that the currently observed increase in hospitalization rate (in several highly vaccinated countries) may simply be the prelude to the big wave of AIESD that I predict will soon sweep through several highly vaccinated populations (chapter 3.4.2.).

3.4.2. Why will highly vaccinated countries not be able to avoid a colossal public health catastrophe?

The steeper the rise in PNNAb-mediated population-level immune pressure, the faster the explosion of cases of enhanced severe disease expected to hit highly vaccinated populations. Depending on vaccine coverage and/or booster rates and/or the type of vaccine and/or vaccination strategy used, I predict that asynchronous waves of AIESD will occur separately in several highly vaccinated countries.

Although it is fair to assume that the first waves of AIESD would start in countries which rapidly and massively vaccinated their population but then largely refrained from repeated booster campaigns[35], I doubt that repeatedly boosted countries' populations will be spared similar "tsunamis" of AIESD for more than a few weeks or months thereafter. Although continued booster doses with the ancestral Wuhan-Hu and/or Omicron-adapted S Ag may *initially* prevent PNNAb titers from declining[36] below the optimal threshold upon re-exposure, there can be no doubt that widespread VBTIs will 'boost' viral uptake into APCs (fig. 11). Recurrent VBTIs will therefore increasingly impede uptake of vaccinal Ag into these cells and prevent recall of CD4+ Th cells. It follows that circulation of highly infectious Omicron descendants is currently causing the immune system of vaccinated individuals to ignore its 'original antigenic sin' as its capacity to further respond to 'calls for recall' rapidly extinguishes.

Even countries/regions that implement extensive infection-prevention measures and quarantines to curtail viral transmission will not be able to prevent or mitigate explosive case fatality rates. This is because highly infectious Omicron variants are now circulating in all highly vaccinated populations and causing vaccinees to exert increasing immune pressure on viral virulence, regardless of their immune status (i.e., due to *Ab-independent* VBTIs). Each highly vaccinated population will now independently breed a SC-variant that dominantly spreads by pairing enhanced viral infectiousness with increased viral virulence (chapter 3.4.1). Each highly vaccinated population is therefore separately planting the seeds for more virulent variants. Surges of severe disease and hospitalization or even waves of AIESD will therefore occur independently in these populations (i.e., regardless of how the virus evolves and spreads in other countries).

Border closures, travel restrictions or isolation of affected regions will therefore not prevent the widespread devastating effect of more virulent immune escape variants.

Given the high level of intrinsic infectiousness of co-circulating Omicron descendants[37] and the increasing 'fatigue' of the host immune system to respond to vaccine booster doses, even the most stringent measures will not suffice to prevent population-level immune pressure on viral virulence from growing ever faster. None of these measures will succeed in mitigating, let alone halting the tsunami of case fatalities. I therefore predict that a multitude of similar waves of AIESD will soon unfold in multiple highly vaccinated countries.

3.5. So far, viral immune escape has not prevented vaccinated individuals from benefiting from protection against severe disease. However, surges in hospitalization[38] rates in several highly vaccinated countries may indicate the beginning of a tsunami of Ab-dependent enhancement of severe disease.

SIR can be triggered by PNNAb-dependent VBTIs caused by EOSVs or by mRNA-based vaccines. SIR is the single most important catalyst of the explosive spread of 'late', highly infectious Omicron descendants. The latter have been reported to incorporate a subset of specific infection-enhancing sequences that converge to S-RBD (ref. 23). Because of their high level of intrinsic viral infectiousness, these new emerging Omicron descendants do not stimulate production of PNNAbs prior to productive infection. Instead, they provoke Ab-independent VBTIs in vaccinated individuals whose CBIIS has not been adequately trained (i.e., because of previously experienced SIR-enabling VBTIs or vaccination with mRNA-based vaccines). However, both PNNAb-dependent and Ab-independent VBTIs provided protection of vaccinated individuals from severe disease.

As the landscape is now monopolized by the new co-circulating variants of high intrinsic infectiousness, highly vaccinated populations are exerting PNNAb-dependent immune pressure on viral *trans* infectiousness and therefore on viral virulence. *Exposure to highly infectious Omicron-derived lineages is now weakening the virulence-neutralizing capacity of PNNAbs in highly vaccinated populations. In other words, Ab-independent VBTIs are now posing the single biggest threat of widespread susceptibility of highly vaccinated populations to an NAb-evasive variant that is capable of breaking through the last hurdle of vaccine-mediated adaptive immune defense (i.e., prevention of severe disease).*

When population-level immune pressure has risen high enough, a majority of vaccinated individuals who did not manage to adequately train their CBIIS could suddenly fall prey to AIESD. However, highly infectious, co-circulating variants that in the meantime have picked up a 'suboptimal' S-associated O-glycosite mutation may propagate while only mitigating protection against severe disease (i.e., becoming more virulent) in individuals with diminished PNNAb-mediated virulence-inhibitory capacity. The higher the PNNAb-mediated immune pressure exerted by the population, the higher the frequency of such cases. It is therefore not surprising that since the advent of highly infectious Omicron-derived variants, several highly vaccinated countries/regions have reported an increasing hospitalization rate. Although these cases are not yet overwhelming the health care system, these surges should, however, be considered the prelude to huge waves of hospitalization and death that I predict will soon unfold independently within several highly vaccinated regions.

3.6. Since exposure to highly infectious Omicron descendants leads to diminished viral shedding, the virus has no choice but to spread within the body of its very host...

Since viral *trans* infection mediates viral *trans* fusion, and since viral *trans* fusion mediates syncytia formation (which is generally considered a correlate for virulence/severe disease), it is fair to conclude that suboptimal immune pressure on viral *trans* infectiousness is equivalent to suboptimal immune pressure on viral virulence. This is now turning highly vaccinated populations into an ideal breeding ground for a new generation of emerging variants capable of blowing through the untrained CBIIS of vaccinated individuals and exhibiting a higher level of virulence *in vivo*.

As a substantial impediment on viral shedding (and therefore on viral transmission to other human hosts) poses a serious threat to survival of the virus, Nature seems to be switching gears. Evolutionary forces reshape virus-host immune interactions in an attempt to secure viral reproduction. By evolving to a higher level of virulence, the virus shifts viral replication and spreads to susceptible organ tissues of the host itself rather than to other susceptible hosts. This leads to a higher mortality rate. During a natural CoV pandemic, case fatalities together with sterilizing immunity developed by the infection-experienced part of the population will ensure reduced viral transmission and thereby speed up herd immunity. Herd immunity terminates the pandemic and subsequently allows asymptomatic viral transmission by immunologically naive individuals (typically, young children). This is how the virus *normally* survives and transitions into endemicity. However, if the virus becomes highly virulent, the survival rate in the population becomes too low for the infection-experienced survivors to ensure a level of viral transmission that is sufficient for the virus to survive. This is why the virus will likely be eradicated when it evolves highly virulent variants as is expected to occur in highly vaccinated countries. Consequently, the mantra spread by health officials and experts that 'we will need to live with the virus' defies the laws of evolutionary biology.

3.7. Training of the CBIIS is no longer possible once a vaccinee experiences a SIR-enabling event. However, some vaccinated individuals will have preserved the capacity to train their CBIIS and will therefore be protected against potentially emerging highly virulent variants to the same extent as the unvaccinated.

SIR-enabling BTIs or mRNA vaccines prevent subsequent training of the CBIIS. SIR-enabling events exclusively occur in vaccinated individuals. As SIR causes the vaccinee's immune system to bypass the CBIIS, and as SIR-enabling VBTIs are triggered by high titers of pNAbs, the only way to prevent vaccination from irreversibly depriving the CBIIS of its training capacity is to train it before vaccine-induced immune priming (in the case of mRNA-based vaccine) or boosting (in the case of non-mRNA-based vaccine) occurs, and to refrain from post-infection vaccination (fig. 1). Deficient or insufficient training of the innate CBIIS will leave vaccinated individuals without any protection when the virus ultimately breaks through the fragile/unstable immune defense that–for now–protects them against (severe) disease.

In the case of mRNA vaccines, the threshold for sidelining the CBIIS is much lower. Based on the mechanism explained in chapters 1.2.1. and 1.2.2., even a single injection of an mRNA vaccine could trigger SIR and abrogate training of the CBIIS if it is administered subsequent to natural infection, even if the latter is asymptomatic (fig. 1).

Since mRNA-based vaccines promote SIR and SIR compromises training of the CBIIS while expediting immune escape in highly vaccinated populations, it seems clear that countries which proceeded with mass vaccination early in the pandemic (i.e., injecting large cohorts prior to natural exposure) and primarily used mRNA vaccines will be the first to fall prey to a massive wave of AIESD. It would not be surprising to find that a high incidence of AIESD could even occur in countries that have relatively low vaccine coverage rates (e.g., < 50%) but only used mRNA-based vaccines. This is because mRNA-based vaccines dramatically expedite immune escape while leaving the CBIIS untrained (except for those who only received a single injection that was not preceded by productive infection (fig. 1)) .

It is interesting to note that the virus can dramatically optimize its immune escape strategy by sidelining the CBIIS. This automatically occurs when insufficient virus-neutralizing capacity prompts PNNAb-dependent VBTIs. Sidelining of the CBIIS enhances the production rate of progeny virus. This is critical to enabling SIR, which accelerates the evolutionary immune escape dynamics of the virus and prevents subsequent training of the CBIIS. mRNA-based vaccines can even trigger SIR in individuals who previously contracted asymptomatic/mild infection.

As exposure to EOSVs could trigger symptomatic PNNAb-mediated BTIs in vaccinated individuals regardless of the training status of their CBIIS, the occurrence of symptomatic VBTI upon exposure to OOV or EOSVs does not inform whether the PNNAb-mediated BTI enabled SIR and therefore prevented future training of their CBIIS. Only PNNAb-mediated BTIs in vaccinated individuals with a sidelined CBIIS enable SIR and therefore have a poor prognosis from both an individual and public health viewpoint (due to irreversible inhibition of cell-based innate immune training and large-scale immune escape respectively). Unfortunately, there is currently no validated assay that allows one to reliably measure the level of cell-based innate immune memory. However, the following categories of vaccinated individuals are still highly likely to have a CBIIS that is sufficiently trained to protect them from highly virulent variants to the same extent as the trained CBIIS of the unvaccinated does (fig. 1):

All healthy vaccinated who had only received a single injection of an mRNA-based vaccine or no more than 2 injections with a non-mRNA-based vaccine prior to developing symptomatic VBTI and who refrained from booster shots after said VBTI.

3.8. Although they occasionally contracted NBTI with early or late Omicron-derived immune escape variants, previously exposed unvaccinated individuals did not experience SIR and can, therefore, rely on their trained CBIIS to prevent productive infection with highly infectious or more virulent Omicron-derived immune escape variants.

Unvaccinated individuals who experienced natural infection with one or more pre-Omicron variants (i.e., in the absence of PNNAbs) developed lower and less durable pNAb titers than those induced by vaccines and trained their CBIIS. The combination of both elements largely prevented the occurrence of PNNAb-mediated NBTIs (fig. 5 panel B).

Nevertheless, unvaccinated individuals occasionally contracted PNNAb-dependent NBTIs as a consequence of rapid reinfection with Omicron after a previous productive infection with a pre-Omicron variant or as a consequence of rapid reinfection with a highly infectious Omicron descendant after a previous productive infection with a EOSV[39]. However, PNNAb-dependent NBTIs in previously exposed unvaccinated individuals were sufficiently dampened by the trained CBIIS in order to prevent a sufficient viral production rate from provoking SIR after rapid re-infection (fig. 5 panel A). Consequently, PNNAb-dependent NBTIs in previously exposed unvaccinated individuals did not trigger SIR and therefore neither drove immune escape nor compromised the CBIIS (fig. 5 panel A and fig. 7). I therefore postulate that the unvaccinated will no longer be susceptible to productive infection with new emerging variants that have at most the same level of intrinsic viral infectiousness (ref. 57) but have a higher level of intrinsic virulence. It is reasonable to assume that individuals who only experienced asymptomatic/mild infection with pre-Omicron variants prior to vaccination with a non-mRNA -based vaccine will be equally well protected from productive infection with new emerging, more infectious or more virulent variants.

However, the likelihood for mRNA-injected vaccinated individuals to experience SIR and hence sideline their CBIIS at an early stage of vaccination is thought to be much higher than in those injected with non-mRNA vaccines. This is because mRNA vaccines can even synergize with asymptomatic/mild infection to enable SIR as of their first post-infection injection. In previously unexposed individuals, a single mRNA vaccine injection can synergize with a single injection of a non-mRNA vaccine to trigger SIR (fig. 1). In other words, the threshold for mRNA vaccines to trigger SIR is much lower than for non-mRNA vaccines. SIR also explains why PNNAb-dependent VBTIs (e.g., upon first exposure of an mRNA-boosted vaccinee to Omicron) cause milder symptoms than PNNAb-dependent NBTIs (e.g., upon first exposure of an unvaccinated person to Omicron shortly after recovery from symptomatic infection).

Sidelining of the CBIIS together with living amongst a highly vaccinated population will dramatically augment the probability for a vaccinated person to succumb to AIESD.

3.9. Natural selection and dominant propagation of Omicron in highly vaccinated populations inevitably exposed these populations to *a series* of abrupt immune pressure-increasing events that *rapidly* resulted in the *co-selection* and *co-circulation* of *several highly infectious immune escape variants*. Highly infectious Omicron descendants are now exposing these populations to a *single* event of *gradually* increasing immune pressure that will take *some time* to *sequentially select* a *single highly virulent* variant (HIVICRON).

Convergence of multiple immune escape mutations in Omicron-derived (sub)variants enabled an important shift in the antigenic and immunologic characteristics of new emerging variants following large-scale PNNAb-dependent BTIs in highly vaccinated populations (i.e., due to incorporation of a shared subset of mutations in more conserved S-RBD and/or S-NTD domains). Hence, dominant circulation of Omicron in highly vaccinated populations drove large-scale immune escape events by fueling widespread SIR-enabling PNNAb-dependent VBTIs (especially in those vaccinated with mRNA-based vaccines).

Whereas large-scale immune pressure on common functional S-associated domains of SIR-enabling VBTIs and/or mRNA booster vaccinations had initially triggered the rapid but temporary[40] reduction of viral infection rates in highly vaccinated populations, these infection rates have gone up again since new, highly infectious immune escape variants emerged. Only a few months after Omicron started to dominate, co-circulation of highly infectious Omicron descendants began prompting highly vaccinated populations to shift their immune pressure on viral infectiousness to immune pressure on viral *trans* infectiousness/virulence (fig. 6).

Exposure of vaccinated individuals to highly infectious co-circulating Omicron descendants is thought to stimulate production of PNNAbs subsequent to Ab-independent VBTI. PNNAb stimulation is likely triggered by pNAb-complexed virions that are not attached to the surface of migratory DCs and cluster into weak aggregates that are subsequently internalized into APCs (thereby enabling CTL-mediated viral clearance) (chapter 3.1.). It is fair to postulate that as long as vaccinal pNAb titers are sufficiently high, the concentration of these Th-independent PNNAbs is collectively increasing upon more widespread exposure or more frequent re-exposure and thereby slowing down the increase in PNNAb-mediated population-level immune pressure on viral virulence. This evolution would explain why it is likely going to take some more time for the virus to select a 'life-saving' immune escape variant capable of dramatically enhancing its intrinsic *trans* infectiousness/virulence.

A more virulent, dominantly circulating variant will likely adapt to the increasing population-level immune pressure generated by Ab-independent VBTIs by incorporating 'more virulent' O-glycosite mutations. It is only when Ab-independent VBTIs combine with decreasing PNNAb titers to fuel population-level immune pressure on viral virulence beyond a threshold sufficient to unleash HIVICRON that a wave of AIESD can be triggered. It is possible that HIVICRON exhibits differences in antigenicity depending on the country/population in which the original, more virulent lineage has been selected to dominantly circulate (e.g., XBB.1.5., chapter 3.4.1.). This, however, should not impact the glycosylation profile or level of virulence of the new, AIESD-enabling variant as the target of the immune pressure exerted by PNNAbs is the *highly conserved* antigenic site within S-NTD,

Whereas PNNAb-dependent VBTIs are followed by a *sudden* increase in population-level immune pressure on intrinsic *viral infectiousness* (after SIR-1 and SIR-2) (fig 6 ❷❸), Ab-independent VBTIs are followed by a *gradual* increase in population-level immune pressure on intrinsic *viral virulence* (i.e., viral trans infectiousness; fig. 6 ❹); the latter is not exerted by *neutralizing* but by *non-neutralizing Abs* (i.e., PNNAbs). Whereas PNNAb-dependent VBTIs promote *co-selection* and -circulation of a diversified subset of highly infectious Omicron-derived [sub]variants, Ab-independent VBTIs promote *sequential* selection of an increasingly virulent Omicron-derived variant, possibly culminating in the selection of a unique highly virulent variant in highly vaccinated populations, herein named HIVICRON.

Chapter Four

Mass vaccination is responsible for the imminent threat to human health. My confidence in the WHO, public health authorities and regulatory bodies is gone. What have they done?

4.1. Highly vaccinated populations exert *herd immune pressure on infectiousness* **instead of generating** *herd immunity against productive infection. Specific humoral immune pressure on viral neutralizability followed by broad humoral immune pressure on viral infectiousness eventually triggered the emergence of co-circulating highly infectious variants* **that now cause highly vaccinated populations to exert humoral immune pressure on viral virulence (figs. 6 and 9).**

Given the following:

> i) Mass vaccination with vaccines during the SC-2 pandemic caused the population to exert suboptimal humoral immune pressure on specific infection-facilitating S-associated domains of the original lineage (i.e., via poorly affinity-matured anti-S Abs) and subsequently on specific neutralizing S-associated domains of the dominantly circulating variant (via affinity-matured anti-S Abs directed at S-RBD);

> ii) Enhanced pNAb-mediated immune pressure on specific neutralizing S-associated domains (i.e., via high-affinity anti-S Abs directed at S-RBD) of the dominantly circulating variant led to rapid natural selection and dominant circulation of an immune escape variant with strongly diminished viral neutralizability (i.e., OOV);

> iii) Dominant circulation of an immune escape variant with strongly diminished viral neutralizability (i.e., OOV) led to an *abrupt* (PNNAb-mediated) increase in viral infectiousness of OOV and therefore caused widespread SIR-enabling VBTIs in highly vaccinated populations;

> iv) Widespread SIR-enabling VBTIs generated an abrupt increase in population-level immune pressure on more conserved neutralizing S-associated domains (i.e., via

broadly neutralizing, low-affinity anti-S Abs induced upon SIR-1) and subsequently on more conserved infection-facilitating S-associated domains (i.e., via broadly infection-inhibiting, low-affinity anti-S Abs induced upon SIR-2);

v) An abrupt increase in population-level immune pressure on more conserved infection-facilitating S-associated domains caused rapid co-emergence and co-circulation of highly infectious Omicron descendants;

vi) Co-circulation of highly infectious Omicron descendants causes a gradual increase in PNNAb-mediated immune pressure on the highly conserved PNNAb-binding domain within S-NTD;

vii) A gradual increase in PNNAb-mediated immune pressure on the highly conserved PNNAb-binding domain within S-NTD promotes sequential selection and dominant propagation of Omicron descendants that pair enhanced intrinsic infectiousness with increasing intrinsic virulence and thereby raise the incidence of severe disease and hospitalizations in vaccinated individuals;

ix) An abrupt and steep increase in PNNAb-mediated immune pressure on the highly conserved PNNAb-binding domain triggers the selection of a highly virulent variant (named 'HIVICRON') capable of provoking widespread cases of AIESD in vaccinated individuals;

Mass vaccination programs implemented during the pandemic are to be blamed for placing vaccinated individuals at high risk of contracting AIESD. As mRNA vaccines trigger SIR, massive deployment of these vaccines has likely expedited immune escape, fostered co-circulation of newly emerging highly infectious variants, and is now raising population-level immune pressure on viral virulence at a pace that may soon dramatically accelerate in several highly vaccinated countries (fig. 9 dotted line in yellow) .

We are left with a dire situation in which the virus will be eradicated and the immune escape pandemic extinguished *only* after unrestrained large-scale AIESD has occurred in highly vaccinated countries. In such countries, all vaccinees deprived of protective CBII (i.e., the majority of a highly vaccinated population) will be at high risk of contracting AIESD or at least severe disease.

4.2. Once the interaction between the virus and the host immune system triggered PNNAb-mediated VBTIs, newly emerging immune escape variants in highly vaccinated populations rapidly accelerated viral immune escape. The latter can now no longer be halted and is doomed to roll all the way to the end station where new emerging variants reach high virulence in those that do not have sufficiently trained CBII.

As the intrinsic infectiousness of circulating Omicron variants has significantly increased and Ab-independent VBTIs are now triggering growing immune pressure on viral virulence, the critical contribution of PNNAbs to propulsing the evolutionary trajectory of the virus has now shifted from *PNNAb-dependent enhancement of viral infectiousness* (i.e., upon emergence of Omicron) to promoting *(PNN)Ab-independent enhancement of severe disease* (i.e., upon pending emergence of a highly virulent variant) [figs. 2, 4, 8 and 9].

Highly vaccinated populations that are exposed to highly infectious Omicron descendants are now relying entirely on PNNAbs to safeguard their protection against severe disease, while paradoxically improving their control of disease symptoms altogether and reducing viral shedding by virtue of enhanced CTL-mediated viral clearance. However, these beneficial effects will come at a price as it's impossible for a highly vaccinated population to further reduce viral shedding of highly infectious Omicron descendants without (gradually) raising PNNAb-mediated immune pressure on viral virulence–both mechanisms are closely linked.

Due to the short half-life of Th-independent PNNAbs, (re-)exposure to *highly*[41] infectious Omicron descendants is the key to maintaining this favorable balance. As the level of PNNAb-mediated inhibition of viral *trans* infectiousness depends on the concentration of PNNAbs, the latter are now collectively exerting suboptimal immune pressure on viral *trans* infectiousness and therefore on viral virulence. Suboptimal immune pressure first fosters immune selection and propagation of more virulent immune escape variants. However, this immune pressure could eventually grow large enough to drive selection and intra-host spread/dissemination of a new variant (i.e., HIVICRON[42]) that is highly resistant to pNAbs and can nullify this pressure thanks to its high level of intrinsic viral virulence.

In the case population-level immune pressure grows steadily but slowly, the threshold necessary to breach the virulence-neutralizing capacity of the PNNAbs in the majority of the vaccinated population may not be reached and a highly virulent variant capable of triggering a large wave of AIESD may not be selected. As already mentioned, this may result in dominant propagation of a more virulent variant that is responsible for an enhanced incidence of severe disease and hospitalizations as already reported in some highly vaccinated countries.

The higher the vaccine coverage rate and vaccine-induced pNAb titers (e.g., as a result of previous vaccine booster doses and/or re-exposure), the stronger the restimulation of PNNAb production following Ab-independent VBTI, and the slower the increase in PNNAb-mediated immune pressure on viral virulence. *The more delayed the increase in immune pressure, the more time it will leave to the virus to produce sufficient progeny necessary to yield a specific variant* endowed with an O-glycosite mutation that can abolish population-level immune pressure by the time such pressure exceeds a threshold sufficient to select a highly virulent variant. As previously mentioned, highly virulent immune escape variants that are antigenically distinct and hit distinct highly vaccinated populations are likely to have incorporated and accommodated the same specific O-glycosite mutation.

Prolonged suboptimal immune pressure on viral virulence is thought to successively select immune escape variants that have acquired and accommodated more elongated O-glycosite mutations enabling a higher level of viral virulence (ref. 5). On the other hand, a steep but delayed rise in immune pressure on viral virulence is likely to instantaneously select the S-associated O-glycosite mutations that will confer a level of virulence sufficient to cause widespread AIESD in the highly vaccinated population (fig. 9 solid and dashed yellow line).

No natural immune mechanisms can be invoked to counter such glycan-based substitutions since saccharidic moieties grafted on the surface of infectious pathogens (e.g., on virus surface-expressed S protein) cannot rely on cognate T help to prime high-affinity memory B cells. However, usage of conjugated glycan-based vaccines in vaccinated individuals is not an option as the conjugated T help Ag will not be able to prime cognate CD4+ T helper cells. This is because the vaccinee's professional APCs at the portal of entry are primarily engaged in stimulating MHC class I-unrestricted CTLs. In other words, no prophylactic conjugated glycan-based vaccine will be able to protect vaccinated individuals as it will fail to induce a neutralizing Ab response against the glycosyl moieties expressed on the S protein of these new variants.

It is reasonable to postulate that as PNNAb-mediated immune pressure collectively exceeds a certain threshold, natural selection of a highly virulent variant that manages to completely lift the immune blockade on viral *trans* infectiousness in the majority vaccinated individuals will be triggered. In the absence of an alternative that specifically protects against viral virulence, the best mechanism to prevent severe disease is a trained CBIIS. As the latter provides sterilizing immunity, it can dramatically reduce viral load at an early stage of infection. A properly trained CBIIS will therefore not only protect against severe disease but even against productive infection *per se*.

Consequently, all vaccinated individuals whose CBII maintenance training has been compromised (for lack or abrogation of training due to a SIR-enabling event) will be highly susceptible to contracting AIESD.

4.3. Have the currently circulating Omicron descendants already become more virulent?

It has already been reported that new emerging Omicron-descendants have higher intrinsic virulence *in vitro* (refs. 48-51). The most likely explanation for this observation is that enhanced viral infectiousness involves changes in the (O-)glycosylation profile of S protein (chapter 3.4.1). However, to the extent that their *in vitro* virulence-enhancing properties are still sufficiently dampened by PNNAbs (*in vivo*), new emerging Omicron-descendants had–until recently–not succeeded in causing widespread VBTIs that led to severe disease. It is therefore reasonable to assume that a new variant that will ultimately be able to trigger enhanced severe disease will be very different (primarily in regard to its [O]-glycosylation profile) from those which have been proven to be more virulent *in vitro*. At the time of this writing (early January 2023) the situation seems to be changing as some highly vaccinated countries (e.g., UK and Ireland) are beginning to see increasing hospitalization rates. This seems to indicate that co-circulating highly infectious variants have begun to translate their enhanced virulence *in vitro* into enhanced virulence *in vivo* and are now well on their way to selecting a highly virulent variant that will manage to bring down the rising population-level immune pressure on viral virulence.

4.4. How will Nature end this immune escape pandemic and restore the profoundly disturbed balance at the benefit of the future generation(s) to come?

In highly vaccinated countries, a high level of viral infectiousness combined with the acquisition of stronger virulence-enhancing properties will likely end with a high incidence of Ab-independent enhancement of severe disease in vaccinated individuals that have no properly trained CBII.

Whereas new emerging highly infectious Omicron descendants have already been shown to be more virulent *in vitro* (refs. 48-51), the incidence of hospitalizations and mortality is–at this time of writing–still fairly low in the majority of highly vaccinated populations. This can only be ascribed to the fact that average pNAb titers in vaccinated individuals are still relatively high and therefore ensure sufficient (re-)stimulation of PNNAbs following Ab-independent VBTI. In other words, sufficiently high concentrations of PNNAbs may–for now–prevent severe disease in the vast majority of vaccinated individuals in highly vaccinated countries . However, it will likely be only a matter of weeks or months before the majority of these populations raise immune pressure on viral virulence to a level necessary to unleash HIVICRON. As soon as this happens, asynchronous waves of vaccine breakthrough cases of enhanced severe disease and death will begin to separately unfold in highly vaccinated countries/regions. This, together with the strong capacity of the unvaccinated to avoid productive infection by co-circulating highly infectious variants (thanks to their adequately trained CBIIS), will likely *eradicate SC-2 and thereby terminate the pandemic.*

It is also probable that large-scale spill-over of a diversified spectrum of variants from animal reservoirs that humans are in contact with and which are protected by herd immunity will ensure prolonged cell-based innate immune training of unvaccinated people (ref. 55). This may help to protect humans from a multitude of other acute self-limiting viral infections. Nature's path to restoring a sound balance between pathogens and the host immune system may provide an exceptional benefit to future generations.

Chapter Five

Research on the immune escape pandemic has become an exercise in mutational stamp collection that does not yield any concrete predictions on the societal impact. Instead, immunological ignorance and mainstream narratives prevail.

5.1. Are scientists no longer seeing the forest for the trees? Why don't they understand that trees have branches (i.e., the glycosyl chains on the spike protein)?

It seems like even the most experienced mutation spotters on this planet are no longer seeing the forest for the trees. Scientists now have access to the most sophisticated technologies for investigating mutational changes in both viral S protein and affinity-maturing Abs. This allows them, for example, to tease out the smallest molecular details of S-associated mutations as the latter evolve in response to the dramatic changes in humoral immune pressure the host immune system is now collectively placing on reproduction and transmission in highly vaccinated populations.

Despite all highly advanced technologies, scientists seem to have forgotten about the basic rules of evolutionary biology. When it comes to a viral immune escape pandemic the latter translate as follows: for as long as an entire population exerts immune pressure on viral *infectiousness* (e.g., on S protein), Nature will select *more infectious* immune escape variants that dominantly or co-dominantly spread (depending on whether population-level immune pressure affects *variable* or more *conserved* epitopes of the protein responsible for infectiousness, respectively). Because enhanced intrinsic viral infectiousness reduces viral shedding, the virus will induce the population to exert immune pressure on viral *trans* infectiousness. Widespread growing immune pressure on viral *trans* infectiousness/*virulence* will eventually lead to the selection of variants exhibiting a *higher level of intrinsic viral virulence* and *capability of provoking severe disease* (i.e., due to viral replication and dissemination in internal organs).

As severe disease (and death) from virulent variants normally occurs in those with a weak or insufficiently trained CBIIS, their natural death normally expedites establishment of herd immunity. The latter sufficiently diminishes viral transmission to prevent symptomatic infection in the population while ensuring viral survival (via some asymptomatic infections). This is how a *natural* pandemic of a virulent virus causing acute self-limiting infection would 'naturally' transition into the endemic state. The critical difference with a pandemic that has evolved highly infectious variants is that widespread growing immune pressure on viral *trans* infectiousness will eventually drive the selection of *more virulent* variants that will rapidly cause an increased incidence of severe disease and even death (due to *enhanced* severe disease). This reflects a profound disturbance of the naturally balanced virus-host immunity ecosystem in which an abrupt and spectacular rise in the occurrence of (enhanced) severe disease will not only inflict an over-proportional damage to the population but also curtail viral transmission to an extent where the virus can no longer survive.

The biggest shortcoming of scientists, regulatory and public health authorities, and even vaccine manufacturers, is that they're unable to grasp that any VBTI (PNNAb-dependent or -independent), or any infection or mRNA booster shot that occurs after a primary series of mRNA vaccinations, or any mRNA vaccination that occurs after previous productive infection (symptomatic or asymptomatic), enables SIR and hence paralyzes the CBIIS while dramatically expediting the immune escape dynamics of the virus.

As they do not understand the concept of SIR, they cannot evaluate the consequences thereof, namely that SIR-mediated immune escape in highly vaccinated populations ultimately leads to a dramatic increase in large-scale, PNNAb-mediated immune pressure on viral virulence. Increasing population-level immune pressure on viral *trans* infectiousness will not stop driving selectional adaptive evolution of S protein *until* it allows the virus to broadly evade the virulence-inhibiting effect exerted by PNNAbs in highly vaccinated populations.

Whereas DMS of the S protein backbone and immunological characterization of pNAbs in sera from infection-inexperienced or convalescent vaccinees allow monitoring of the evolutionary dynamics of immune pressure on viral neutralizability and infectiousness, mutational scanning of O-linked glycosylation patterns and immunological characterization of PNNAbs in sera from vaccinees could provide insight on the evolutionary dynamics of immune pressure on viral virulence. As this type of data are not currently available, my predictions in regard to the likelihood for virulence-enhancing mutations to occur are largely based on the putative molecular mechanism of PNNAb-mediated inhibition of viral trans infectiousness as investigated in vitro and on the molecular understanding of why and how selection of O-glycosite mutations with more extensive glycosylation enable SC-2 to adapt to enhanced PNNAb-mediated immune pressure on viral virulence.

Whereas key opinion leaders and health experts seem to be confident that SC-2 is becoming less pathogenic and in the process of transitioning into endemicity, I am predicting that a new, more infectious and highly virulent immune escape variant ('HIVICRON')[43] will result in massive, separately developing waves of AIESD in several distinct highly vaccinated populations.

In the meantime, I postulate that the mutational S-associated changes required to unlock viral trans infectiousness in vaccinated individuals will not affect the protection the unvaccinated have established against highly infectious variants thanks to maintenance training of their CBII. Irrespective of enhanced intrinsic infectiousness of the virus, the trained CBIIS of the unvaccinated will successfully eliminate virus-infected cells at an early stage of infection and therefore protect from symptomatic infection.

5.2. Productive infection with infectious virus in the absence of both NAbs and a trained CBIIS *promotes severe disease.* **However, exposure of vaccinated individuals to more infectious viruses in the presence of pNAbs lacking sufficient neutralizing capacity** *promotes protection against severe disease.* **In highly vaccinated populations, PNNAb-dependent VBTIs and mRNA booster doses initially provided short-lived protection against productive infection and subsequently** *prolonged protection against disease.* **This is why society, including the medical community, will be caught by surprise when all of a sudden HIVICRON will provoke widespread enhancement of severe disease in highly vaccinated parts of the world.**

The different outcome of exposure of 'untrained' individuals to infectious virus in the absence of NAbs and a trained CBIIS as compared to those with high titers of pNAbs lacking sufficient neutralizing capacity can be explained by the role of PNNAbs. These Abs recognize a highly conserved NTD-associated enhancing site that is comprised within S-NTD (refs. 2-4); they are short-lived, polyreactive and Th-independent and only elicited in the presence of relatively high concentrations of poorly neutralizing Abs. I therefore hypothesize that these Abs are elicited by multimeric arrays of the conserved, immunocryptic NTD-associated enhancing site. Such arrays are thought to be expressed on pNAb-SC-2 complexes that cluster as small viral aggregates.

As PNNAbs in vaccinated individuals can trigger VBTIs and as PNNAb-dependent VBTIs provoke a high production rate of progeny virus, it is reasonable to assume that pNAbs will no longer bind in sufficient concentration to S protein expressed on the surface of progeny virions to ensure rapid internalization into professional APCs (chapter 1.2.3.). Instead, binding of pNAbs would lead to steric masking of immunodominant S-associated epitopes and thereby trigger SIR. SIR is a salient feature in vaccinated individuals who experience post-vaccination infections with heterologous variants (i.e., variants that are decorated with an S protein variant that is antigenically very different from the ancestral Wuhan-Hu S protein used in the vaccine).

SIR-enabling VBTIs (and SIR-enabling mRNA vaccinations) allow for short-lived protection against productive infection (i.e., via *de novo* priming of new, broadly functional anti-S Abs of low affinity (chapters 1.2.4. and 1.2.7.)) but eventually drive the emergence of new immune escape variants. As the latter are equipped with the same immunodominant S-associated epitopes, they maintain the ability to bind to high concentrations of vaccinal pNAbs[44] and trigger re-stimulation of Th-independent PNNAbs. The latter will provide protection against severe disease in vaccinated individuals regardless of whether their production resulted from PNNAb-dependent or (PNN)Ab-independent VBTI.

Following VBTI with highly infectious Omicron descendants, enhanced capture of free progeny virions by vaccinal pNAbs will occur and facilitate abundant uptake of highly infectious progeny virions into tissue-resident APCs. This strengthens the host's cytolytic attack on virus-infected cells and not only diminishes viral shedding but also attenuates disease symptoms in vaccinated individuals.

In summary, as described above in chapters 1.2.10. and 3.1., massive VBTIs in vaccinated individuals caused by highly infectious co-circulating variants entails dilution of the concentration of PNNAbs adsorbed to DC-tethered virions and (re-)stimulates the production of these Abs (especially in vaccinated individuals with high [i.e.,boosted!] vaccinal pNAb titers). This causes highly vaccinated populations to only gradually augment PNNAb-mediated immune pressure on viral *trans* infectiousness/viral virulence while revving up elimination of virus-infected cells. It is therefore not surprising that while the virus is now preparing for the elicitation of Ab-independent enhancement of severe disease in vaccinated individuals, more and more vaccinated individuals seem to be benefiting from enhanced mitigation of disease symptoms.

That's why I am predicting that society in highly vaccinated countries will be caught by surprise.

I expect that gradually increasing hospitalization rates already observed in some highly vaccinated countries are only the prelude to gigantic, separately developing waves of deaths that will first and foremost affect countries/regions that rapidly proceeded with mass immunization of their population using mRNA-based vaccines and repeated booster doses. As highly infectious Omicron descendants do not induce SIR-enabling VBTIs and exclusively drive viral immune escape by enhancing population-level immune pressure on viral virulence, it seems likely that differences in the outcome of viral immune escape between different highly vaccinated countries/regions will soon be limited to distinct time-points of the respective onsets of enhanced hospitalization rates and delayed explosions in the mortality rates. I therefore predict that– on a global scale– circulation of highly infectious Omicron descendants will eventually translate into a single "mega wave" of death that spreads across several highly vaccinated regions, and that this mega wave will likely last for only a few months before ending the immune escape pandemic in those countries.

5.3. Why don't the mutation spotters ring the alarm bell?

Given the level of concern raised by the enhanced evolutionary dynamics of Omicron variants, I am profoundly disappointed by the interpretations and conclusions of molecular epidemiologists 'watching' the current explosion of new emerging Omicron variants. None of their conclusions have substantial predictive value for individual or global health; they are mostly featured by *ad hoc* interpretations that no longer apply to subsequent emerging variants. Their conclusions are therefore of no use to society (e.g., 'the immune responses currently elicited by prolonged or repeated exposure to S antigen will likely continue to impact the future course and pace of SARS-CoV-2 variant emergence while contributing to ongoing vaccine-mediated protection against severe disease' or 'deep mutational scanning datasets [on Omicron-derived variants] identify shifts in the mutational landscape and inform ongoing efforts in viral surveillance').

Massive exercises in mutational stamp collection combined with *ad hoc* interpretations of the resulting data have been the biggest obstacle for scientists to acknowledge the disastrous consequences of this mass vaccination experiment; their mutational analyses and predictive epidemiological modeling merely reflect snapshots and don't consider the immunological dynamics that are driving natural selection of suitable mutations.

Notwithstanding the fact that the vast majority of authors admit they don't understand the underlying causes of the evolving host immune pressure, they also don't seem to have any reservation when it comes to advocating for more mass vaccination (e.g., 'understanding the evolution of Ab immunity following heterologous breakthrough infection will inform the development of next-generation vaccines'; 'Monitoring the rapidly evolving epidemiological landscape and newly emerging variants is of high importance for guiding vaccine adaptation programs')

5.4. The pandemic landscape in highly vaccinated countries is currently dominated by a formidable expansion of more infectious viral immune escape variants that–instead of generating herd immunity–are now paving the way to a global health catastrophe. In the meantime our leading scientists and health experts seem to be suffering from immunological ignorance and willful blindness.

Global health authorities, key opinion leaders, health experts and scientists all relentlessly supported or even drove the mainstream narrative preaching that the spread of circulating Omicron variants would be a blessing and would boost vaccine-induced immunity. This combined with their more benign disease phenotype would rapidly herald the transition of this pandemic into endemicity. This is fundamentally wrong–there isn't even a need to take a deep dive in the underlying immunological mechanisms to understand that the evolutionary dynamics of this immune escape pandemic do not comply with this viewpoint:

❖ Instead of reducing the viral infection and transmission rate (as is the case with herd immunity established upon *mass immunization* during a natural pandemic), *mass vaccination* campaigns initially resulted in an enhanced viral infection rate and more recently in the emergence of new highly infectious variants that escaped from neutralizing S-directed Abs. Steadily increasing infection rates and the evolution of higher intrinsic infectiousness are both phenomena that have never been observed during a natural pandemic. There is simply no evidence of any viral pandemic that bred dominantly or co-dominantly circulating variants that increasingly evaded previously primed NAbs; all of this argues against herd immunity being established.

➤ To put it bluntly: to pretend that an *immune escape pandemic* could generate herd immunity is a *contradictio in terminis*.

➢ As no herd immunity has been established, the pandemic cannot transition into endemicity.

However, there have been several different publications that report clear-cut proof of immune responses in vaccinated individuals being escaped by a multiplicity of rapidly emerging variants with enormous propagation advantage (ref. 28). Although these reports are corroborating the invalidity of the "endemicity fairy tale", none of them provide a scientific/rational explanation on why SC-2 has evolved from selecting specific variants that evade specific virus-neutralizing Abs in vaccinated individuals to promoting co-circulation of several new immune escape variants that independently acquired identical mutations to accomplish a high level of intrinsic infectiousness (fig. 9).

Although scientists seem to agree that convergent evolution of mutations to a well-defined subdomain of S protein (be it the S-RBD- or S-NTD-associated antigenic domain) is driven by *population-level immune selection pressure* placed on the virus, none of them dares to mention what's become crystal clear: the evolutionary dynamics of the virus have only been accelerated and the diversity of the mutational landscape expanded shortly after substantial parts of the population were vaccinated (during the pre-Omicron phase), and especially so since booster doses dramatically expanded the prevalence of VBTIs (since the advent of Omicron).

It would be interesting to compare viral evolutionary dynamics in highly vaccinated countries (with similar vaccine coverage rates across the vaccinated age groups) that exclusively used non-mRNA-based vaccines with those that exclusively used mRNA-based vaccines–there is compelling mechanistic evidence that SIR-enabling mRNA-based vaccines greatly expedite immune escape.

In addition, no scientist seems to understand that the ongoing evolutionary trajectory of this virus is threatening mankind with an unprecedented major but immunosilent (glycan-based) shift that will likely evolve a highly virulent variant (HIVICRON) in widely vaccinated populations. Based on scientifically sound and compelling immunological principles, I have explained how S protein in NAb-

evasive variants could incorporate additional glycosyl moieties at mutated O-glycosites to weaken or even fully break through the virulence-inhibiting effect of PNNAbs, thereby causing AIESD in vaccinated individuals with an untrained or insufficiently trained CBIIS. As PNNAb-mediated immune pressure in highly vaccinated populations is growing, the question is not if but when this will happen.

To investigate the credibility of the mainstream narrative, it would probably suffice to have our leading scientists and health experts address the following questions (all of which have been extensively addressed in the chapters above)

❖ *Why did hospitalization and mortality rates no longer follow high infection rates after the advent of Omicron? How can this disconnect be explained?*

❖ *Initially, vaccinal pNAbs protected against disease. Although recently emerging Omicron descendants are highly infectious and now largely or even fully resistant to pNAbs, more vaccinated individuals are now experiencing mitigation of disease symptoms. Why?*

No scientist seems to have an explanation as to why the strongly diminished neutralizing capacity of pNAbs against EOSVs, or the enhanced intrinsic viral infectiousness and lack of neutralizability of the currently circulating Omicron-derived variants, have not resulted in higher hospitalization or mortality rates, but rather led to even lower morbidity and mortality rates overall (as explained above, it's only quite recently that this trend has started to change in some highly vaccinated countries).

In other words, nobody seems to understand how enhanced susceptibility to early Omicron infection or enhanced intrinsic viral infectiousness of new emerging Omicron descendants can be reconciled with prevention of severe disease or even disease symptoms altogether in vaccinated individuals whose Abs no longer possess (sufficient) neutralizing capacity.

There are also other "anomalies" none of our leading scientists seem to be able to explain, i.e., the sudden disconnect between the high viral infection rate and age (as high incidence of infection is no longer limited to the elderly) and season (a high infection rate occurred during the summer of 2022).

As explained above, even their conclusion that highly vaccinated populations have now reached herd immunity is entirely wrong.

It's no wonder that the contribution of PNNAbs to inhibiting viral virulence as a final obstacle to a health catastrophe is not understood by those who blindly believe the virus will never remove this hurdle for risk of jeopardizing its very existence–but viruses don't "think". If this were true, a virus would not even consider starting an infection in an immunologically naïve and predominantly immunocompromised population (e.g., elderly, those with underlying diseases or otherwise immune suppressed). As most in this population would lack sufficient cell-based innate immune capacity and adequately matched adaptive immunity, the majority would be killed for lack of functional immunity and cause the virus to be eradicated for lack of susceptible hosts. *However, we know that the virus would not take this into account.*

Regardless of the astonishing lack of understanding and insight, many scientists also seem to blindly endorse the proposal of incompetent health authorities and dubious public health experts to continue the mass vaccination experiment with Omicron-adapted mRNA-based vaccines. Not understanding that Omicron-adapted booster doses only expedite(d) immune escape and fail to prime new neutralizing Abs towards the updated S sequence is probably one of the most blatant examples of their immunological ignorance.

In summary, it seems like none of those who are currently supporting or even dictating the mainstream narrative and/or providing 'scientific' advice to our governing bodies understand that we're currently in a calm before the imminent tsunami, and that the *temporary* benefit of the mass vaccination experiment on (severe) disease will soon revert itself into an unprecedented public health disaster in highly vaccinated countries.

5.5. Even scientists dedicated to the pandemic do not seem to understand that a steady increase in large-scale immune pressure on viral virulence will eventually promote natural selection of an Omicron descendant that has picked up a highly virulent mutation. Selection of a new variant of this sort poses an imminent threat of an unprecedented health catastrophe in highly vaccinated countries, yet several scientists continue to pretend that the situation is under control and that protection against severe disease is durable and largely relies on cross-reactive memory T cells.

It is surprising that several scientists continue to pretend that protection of vaccinated individuals against severe disease is long-lived as they consider this protection largely the result of cross-reactive *memory* T cells. First, it is difficult to understand how cross-reactive memory T cells in vaccinated individuals would only occasionally protect against severe disease (e.g., in the case of PNNAb-dependent VBTIs) and occasionally against disease symptoms altogether (e.g., in the case of PNNAb-independent VBTIs). Such a divergence in functionality of cross-reactive memory T cells elicited within a single individual has not been previously reported. If cross-reactive *memory* T cells were the responsible mechanism of protection, individuals who recovered from previous symptomatic infection would be protected from future symptomatic infection (which is indeed not the case as several individuals who fully recovered from previous symptomatic infection with pre-Omicron variants experienced another occurrence of disease upon subsequent exposure to Omicron).

If the origin of prolonged, large-scale immune protection from a disease that is caused by an acute self-limiting viral infection (e.g., CoV) were to be sought in T cell-mediated protective immunity, it would have to rely on cross-reactive memory T cells that are endowed with cytotoxic capacity towards all antigenic variants, regardless of the MHC haplotypes of the host. Regardless of whether these MHC-unrestricted T cells were induced by natural productive infection or vaccination, they would be expected to durably prevent disease (not just *severe* disease) as of the first (re-) exposure to SC-2. However, this cannot be reconciled with the occurrence of symptomatic BTIs in both unvaccinated and vaccinated individuals after previous recovery from disease or previous vaccination respectively. If cytotoxic T memory cells were responsible for recovery from disease, one could not explain why VBTIs with OOV or EOSVs only provided short-lived protection from disease upon re-exposure.

If such cross-reactive cytolytic *memory* T cells were generated during the evolutionary course of an immune escape pandemic, we would at least find *some* evidence amongst the countless publications on infection- or vaccine-induced T cell immunity that either natural infection or vaccination can induce those cells. Such evidence is, however, not available.

Lastly, recently published evolutionary changes in MHC class I-restricted Tc epitopes of Omicron descendants are *not* proof of T cell involvement in viral control either (refs. 46, 47, 58). This is because evolution is not always driven by natural selection but may also result from non-selectional adaptive evolution or stochastic co-evolution (ref. 10). This occurs, for example, when a population specifically adapts to a situation without causing any difference in the reproductive value between the specific genotypes. In the case of SC-2 for example, one could easily imagine that genetic differences stochastically occur among naturally selected genotypes in parts of the viral genome that are not under immune selection pressure. One should not conclude that all immunogenetic differences between circulating variants are due to *natural immune selection* and therefore reflect immune escape.

It would take some experimental work to find out whether specific different immunogenetic traits simply co-evolved with selectional adaptive evolution of other traits or whether they are selectional on their own. It is only when immunogenetic traits can be unambiguously associated with systematic differences in the reproductive value between the corresponding variants that one can conclude them a result of immune selection pressure. As far as Tc epitopes are concerned, there is no immunological evidence or immunopathogenic mechanisms suggesting that Tc epitopes are under population-level immune pressure.

Taken together, it is fair to conclude that the type of immune response that provides *prolonged* protection against (severe) disease cannot be based on memory T cells and is therefore *not durable*.

THE INESCAPABLE IMMUNE ESCAPE PANDEMIC

5.6. The scientific community agrees that convergent evolution of 'concerning' immune escape variants in highly vaccinated populations results from population-level immune selection pressure placed on the virus. Why does no one investigate the origin of this population-level immune pressure?

Reports on convergent evolution of mutations in new emerging variants offer a unique but yet unexploited opportunity to identify the origin and nature of humoral immune pressure that highly vaccinated populations are placing on viral infectiousness and how this immune pressure is evolving in parallel with the evolutionary dynamics of the virus (figs. 6 and 9).

It is truly astonishing that none of these studies even suggests immune refocusing as a major element in driving convergent evolution of mutations in more conserved, S-associated antigenic domains. No one has been exploring the underlying mechanism responsible for the profound and rapidly occurring changes that have been observed in the functional capacity of the elicited anti-S Abs since Omicron became the dominant lineage. Nobody has been investigating the immune correlates of expedited large-scale immune escape that materialized in the rapid co-circulation of several antigenically distinct Omicron descendants that evolved to share the same immune-evasive mutations.

Chapter Six

Even if the road is bumpy, a naturally trained CBIIS is the (only) key to protection from viral immune escape variants and to taming a viral immune escape pandemic.

6.1. In contrast to vaccine-primed immunity, adaptive immune priming by natural infection is dampened by the CBIIS. Vaccinated individuals acquired protection from disease caused by pre-Omicron through vaccine-induced NAbs whereas the unvaccinated acquired such protection through a combination of trained CBIIS and NAbs. However, this immune protection did not suffice to protect either group from BTIs with Omicron. However, trained CBII in the unvaccinated prevented these BTIs from enabling SIR.

PNNAb-dependent BTIs can occur upon SC-2 exposure in the presence of Abs that have insufficient neutralizing capacity, whether resulting from previous vaccination or natural infection. However, productive infection in healthy individuals enables training of innate immune killer cells (i.e., trained Natural Killer [NK] cells), the functional reprogramming of which promotes rapid elimination of virus-infected host cells upon subsequent re-exposure to the same viral lineage. Productive infections that cannot be readily controlled by the CBIIS prime NAbs. Such post-infection NAbs synergize with trained CBII to enable sterilizing immunity upon subsequent re-exposure with the same viral lineage or to protect against disease in case of exposure to a sufficiently neutralizable viral *variant*. Re-exposure of previously infected individuals to the circulating virus or a slightly different variant recalls high titers of previously infection-primed NAbs which contribute to protection against disease. However, this protection mechanism has its limits–recalled NAbs may not sufficiently neutralize a new, more infectious variant to prevent disease. This is why previous infection with a more distant pre-Omicron variant did not always provide reliable protection from exposure to the more infectious Delta variant, especially if the previous infection only provoked mild symptoms.

However, with the advent of Omicron, lack of protection against infection became much more generalized even in those who previously experienced symptomatic disease. Because of the spectacular changes in its S-RBD, OOV was no longer sufficiently neutralizable by the infection-primed NAbs. Furthermore, NAb titers had meanwhile risen to high levels in a substantial part of the unvaccinated population due to (re-)exposure to more infectious pre-Omicron immune escape variants. High concentrations of pre-existing, poorly neutralizing Abs could therefore bind in sufficiently high concentrations to OOV's S protein and thereby trigger clustering of the virus into weak aggregates expressing multimeric arrays of S-NTD-associated Th-independent Ag at their surface. As this is thought to stimulate production of PNNAbs, dominant circulation of Omicron likely rendered a substantial part of the unvaccinated population susceptible to PNNAb-dependent NBTI (fig. 5 panel A).

This would explain why a substantial part of the healthy unvaccinated population suddenly contracted disease (while being granted PNNAb-mediated protection from severe symptoms) when exposures to OOV expanded in prevalence. However, since a trained first line of immune defense (i.e., CBIIS) has the capacity to mitigate the production rate of progeny virus, it is reasonable to assume that high pNAb titers in those who experienced NBTI exceeded the available concentration of progeny virions and therefore enhanced CTL-mediated viral clearance rather than triggering SIR (fig. 5 panel A) (chapter 3.1.). This would also explain why–thanks to training of their CBIIS–the unvaccinated did not contribute to viral immune escape and were not responsible for turning this pandemic into an *immune escape pandemic.*

Based upon the putative mechanism explained above, it is not surprising that disease in unvaccinated individuals primarily occurred in those who became exposed to OOV or EOSVs shortly (i.e., within 4 to 6 weeks) after previous pre-Omicron infection (e.g., with the Delta variant; fig. 5 panel A). Dominant circulation of more infectious pre-Omicron variants led to an increased infection rate and therefore increased the likelihood of re-exposure to a new variant shortly after previous productive infection. The same phenomenon likely occurred–though less frequently[45]–when an unvaccinated person who previously recovered from OOV or EOSV became exposed to a highly infectious Omicron descendant shortly after his/her recovery. This is because highly infectious Omicron descendants have incorporated a subset of new mutations in their S-RBD.

Exposure in the presence of pre-existing Abs (i.e., shortly after previous exposure to a more distant Omicron-derived variant) may even have enhanced the susceptibility of some unvaccinated individuals to pulmonary disease caused by other respiratory pathogens. This can be explained by *in vitro* studies showing viral sensing creates an inflammatory environment that promotes lectin-mediated *trans* infection. Although PNNAb-dependent NBTIs do not induce SIR (fig. 5 panel A) , NBTIs caused by highly infectious Omicron descendants likely generated a more inflammatory environment by boosting the viral production rate. This would promote upregulation of lectin expression on DCs and thereby favor attachment of highly infectious progeny virus onto their membrane (rather than internalizing it) (ref. 40). Attachment of viral particles to DCs facilitates viral *trans* infectiousness. Subsequent migration of these cells to the LRT may therefore facilitate *trans* infection of SC-2 virions to lung epithelial cells. While this didn't seem to trigger systemic virus dissemination, it generated a more inflammatory environment in the lungs. This would explain why exposure to highly infectious Omicron descendants has been provoking secondary bacterial infection and respiratory symptoms in some unvaccinated individuals, especially in those with underlying pulmonary disease or hypersensitivities.

However, in the vast majority of unvaccinated individuals, exposure to these more infectious immune escape variants further contributed to training of their CBIIS and elicit at most some mild disease symptoms (but not PNNAb-dependent BTI).

As the vaccines used for the mass vaccination program do not use replicating viruses and therefore do not allow for training of the CVIIS, vaccinated individuals had to rely exclusively on their vaccinal Abs to acquire protection against disease. As vaccines induce much higher NAb titers than natural infection does[46] (with the exception of natural infections causing severe disease), the majority of the vaccinated acquired NAb titers that were high enough to protect them from new, more infectious pre-Omicron variants[47] that dominantly circulated in highly vaccinated populations. However, that situation suddenly changed with the advent of Omicron. Akin to the situation of the unvaccinated, vaccinees equipped with high titers of poorly neutralizing Abs became highly susceptible to PNNAb-dependent BTIs (fig. 5 panel C). The latter therefore primarily occurred in vaccinated individuals who became exposed to Omicron after having received a non-mRNA vaccine injection subsequent to symptomatic infection or as a booster dose.

In the case of irreversible sidelining of the CBIIS by a previous SIR event, the production rate of progeny virus generated upon PNNAb-mediated VBTI cannot be mitigated. It is therefore reasonable to assume that the concentration of progeny virions in vaccinated individuals who experienced VBTI exceeded the available concentration of pNAb titers and therefore triggered SIR rather than enhancing CTL-mediated viral clearance (see chapters 1.2.3. and 2.2.). SIR drives the host immune system to refocus on other subdominant S-associated domains and therefore promotes widespread VBTIs upon exposure to OOV. It is therefore reasonable to assume that sidelining of the CBIIS in vaccinated individuals enabled EOSVs to trigger rapid and large-scale immune escape in highly vaccinated populations (fig. 5 panels C and D) (fig.7). This strongly suggests that since the advent of Omicron, vaccinated individuals have been a breeding ground for *large-scale* immune escape in highly vaccinated populations and were responsible for turning this pandemic into an *inescapable immune escape pandemic.*

It should be highlighted that even an immune system that has been properly primed by natural infection with a pre-Omicron variant can still be subject to SIR. The immune system of previously SC-2-infected individuals can therefore still be taught to refocus on other subdominant S-associated domains. Infection-experienced individuals could therefore still contribute to promoting large-scale immune escape instead of continuing training of their innate immune cells. This is, for example, the case when non-mRNA-based vaccines are administered to individuals who previously recovered from symptomatic infection or when mRNA-based vaccines are used in previously infection-primed individuals. Based on immunological considerations (chapters 1.2.1. and 1.2.2.), it is plausible that mRNA-based vaccines not only trigger SIR in previously vaccine-primed individuals but also in previously infection-primed individuals[48]. This is because mRNA-based vaccines on their own, or in combination with natural infection, are prone to trigger SIR (figs. 1, 5 panel D and 7).

This would strongly suggest that mRNA-based mass vaccination caused massive abrogation of cell-based innate immune training in highly vaccinated populations (figs. 1 and 4). As SIR also promotes large-scale PNNAb-mediated VBTIs, SIR-enabling vaccines (i.e., mRNA-based vaccines) irreversibly sideline cell-based innate immune training and expedite large-scale immune escape.

In conclusion, during the pre-Omicron phase of this immune escape pandemic, the majority of healthy unvaccinated and the majority of the vaccinated[49] were protected from disease whereas a substantial part of both groups lost this protection upon exposure to Omicron. However, whereas loss of protection led to SIR-enabling VBTIs in vaccinated individuals, trained CBII in the unvaccinated prevented NBTIs from provoking SIR. Consequently, vaccinated individuals, but not the unvaccinated, have been a breeding ground for large-scale immune escape since the advent of Omicron.

6.2. Enhanced intrinsic infectiousness of immune escape variants diminishes viral shedding. As viral infectiousness of newly emerging (more virulent) immune escape variants does no longer increase, trained CBII in the unvaccinated can catch up with new emerging variants to protect the unvaccinated from symptomatic infection. Sterilizing immunity in the unvaccinated combined with a high mortality rate in the vaccinated will eventually lead to natural extinction of the pandemic in highly vaccinated populations.

Because naturally induced Abs suffer as much from the immune-evasive properties of the virus as the vaccinal Abs, the only chance for those caught up in a viral immune escape pandemic to control circulating viral immune escape variants is to train their variant-nonspecific CBII. This is because CBII can be trained to adapt to the evolving level of viral infectiousness that results due to immune escape of the virus.

A 'trained' CBIIS (i.e., equipped with innate cell-based memory) is very efficient with MHC-unrestricted killing of virus-infected cells at an early stage of infection. In case of a natural pandemic, large-scale induction of infection-primed NAbs together with trained CBII enables large-scale sterilizing immunity and entails a drastic reduction of viral transmission in the population. As soon as the viral transmission rate has fallen low enough, herd immunity will be established and the natural pandemic will terminate. In other words, *large-scale natural immunity is required and sufficient to protect an individual from a pandemic virus and to end a natural pandemic* (of an acute self-limiting infection). This, however, implies that the majority of the population is capable of training their CBIIS. However, mass vaccination during a natural pandemic turns the pandemic into an immune escape pandemic and drives the vaccinated into sidelining their CBIIS. The latter is therefore unable to be trained to adapt to immune escape variants that evolve to evade neutralizing Abs and become more infectious. It is therefore not surprising that in the case of an immune escape pandemic, the road for both the unvaccinated individual and the overall population to acquire protection from the evolving virus is treacherous.

First, the diminished neutralization capacity of pNAbs in individuals who previously experienced productive infection may enable the virus to bypass the CBIIS, thereby causing symptomatic PNNAb-mediated NBTIs (see above). However, as the pandemic evolves and viral infectiousness grows, viral shedding of the Omicron-derived immune escape variants diminishes (see chapters 3.2. and 3.3.). If the negative impact of reduced shedding on viral transmission outweighs the positive impact of enhanced viral infectiousness, the frequency of PNNAb-mediated NBTIs will diminish. This may explain why the unvaccinated are now less likely to contract disease.

Finally, the virus is likely to evolve more virulent lineages through glycosylated mutations. However, glycosylation of S protein does not involve enhancement of intrinsic viral infectiousness (ref. 57). Hence, there is no need for unvaccinated[50] individuals, whose CBIIS received the latest training instructions following exposure to co-circulating highly infectious variants, to further adapt to a higher level of viral infectiousness to control these new emerging, more virulent variants. In other words, the unvaccinated will ultimately acquire full-fledged protection from disease. They may even be largely protected from productive infection. This protection will be solely conferred by their trained CBIIS.

However, the population in highly vaccinated countries/regions will face a bumpy road as well because herd immunity will not be established for lack of insufficient collective immune sterilizing capacity. This is because the latter is primarily conferred by the unvaccinated part of the population which–in highly vaccinated countries/regions–is the minority of the population. It is only when mortality rates spectacularly rise in the part of the population that will fail to control co-circulating highly infectious variants growing more virulent (i.e., exclusively comprising the vaccinated) that the level of viral transmission will eventually fall low enough to cause spontaneous extinction of the virus and thereby end the pandemic (chapters 3.4. and 4.4.).

In summary, it is reasonable to conclude that only large-scale natural immunity will tame a natural or immune escape pandemic. In the case of a natural pandemic, both large-scale trained CBII and small-scale priming of humoral adaptive immunity will enable the population to end the pandemic (via herd immunity). In an immune escape pandemic, small-scale trained CBII (in the unvaccinated) by itself will not suffice to end the pandemic. Nature will therefore need to provide an additional tool to curtail viral transmission in order to terminate the pandemic. The tool under development is called large-scale 'Ab-independent enhancement of viral virulence'. It is clear that this 'tool' will be developed in the majority of the population that cannot control the virus through trained CBII (i.e., vaccinated individuals) and thereby exerts growing immune pressure on viral replication/transmission.

Chapter Seven

Omicron and mRNA vaccines– or the combination of both– are a public health scourge, not a blessing.

7.1. Steric immune refocusing (SIR) is not only a hallmark of PNNAb-mediated VBTIs with Omicron but also of mRNA booster immunizations–both drive large-scale and diversified immune escape

As Omicron exhibits substantial NAb evasion, it is prone to stimulating T help-independent PNNAbs that bind to SC-2 and render it more infectious. Following PNNAb-dependent VBTIs, masking of immunodominant S protein-derived epitopes occurs as a result of their weak binding to previously vaccine-primed pNAbs. Because the latter are a poor match to the heterologous S variant, they only bind with low affinity and can therefore not outcompete hACE2 for binding to the S-RBD. Exposure of the immunodominant S-associated epitopes to these pre-existing S-specific Abs is likely to refocus the newly elicited Abs to the subdominant domains of S protein. With the help of bystander memory Th cells, the resulting breakthrough infections enable priming of low affinity anti-S Abs that are directed at subdominant, S-associated epitopes expressed on the surface of free circulating S protein (released from infected cells). This is how PNNAb-mediated VBTIs with Omicron refocused the immune response towards more conserved S-associated antigenic domains.

Booster doses of mRNA-based vaccines also likely enable masking of immunodominant S protein-derived epitopes. In the case of mRNA vaccines, these epitopes are masked by low-affinity anti-S Abs that were previously primed by the mRNA vaccine itself. Since the recalled anti-S Abs have low affinity, a diversified spectrum of functional immune responses has been observed in sera from convalescent vaccinated individuals or in those who received an mRNA booster dose or were exposed after a primary series of mRNA vaccine shots, or who received an mRNA vaccine dose after productive infection (refs. 21-32).

Large-scale PNNAb-enabling VBTIs and mRNA vaccinations likely generated a continuum of immune responses with differential functional capacity towards newly emerging variants (ref. 28) while ensuring a gradual increase in population-level immune pressure on the overall neutralizability and infectiousness of SC-2 virus.

However, regardless of all analytical complexity, it is obvious that since the advent of Omicron all evolutionary scenarios in highly vaccinated populations converged to large-scale viral immune escape and gave rise to a more diversified spectrum of co-circulating Omicron-derived immune escape variants (fig. 9).

7.2. mRNA booster shots (including Omicron-updated mRNA boosters) promoted SIR and therefore expedited immune escape in triple mRNA-vaccinated individuals. However, given the emergence of new highly infectious Omicron descendants, immune escape in highly vaccinated populations is no longer driven by SIR but solely dependent on Ab-independent VBTIs

Immune responses elicited by booster doses using updated Omicron-adapted mRNA formulations, including bivalent formulations of the original Moderna and Pfizer mRNA SARS-CoV-2 vaccines, [51] were short-lived and did not induce superior neutralizing antibody responses in humans compared to the original monovalent mRNA vaccine formulation, nor did they elicit significant titers of Omicron variant-specific Abs (refs. 36-39) . This seems to confirm that–alike previous mRNA booster doses–updated Omicron-adapted mRNA booster doses only induced low-affinity memory B cells towards more conserved, subdominant S-associated epitopes. Consequently, these large-scale immunizations primarily generated high immune pressure on more conserved S protein-associated sites[52].

As immune re-focusing prevents boosting of pNAbs directed at Omicron-specific immunodominant epitopes while enhancing the immunogenicity of only a limited subset of more conserved subdominant antigenic determinants, it narrows the humoral Ab repertoire instead of diversifying it (ref. 23). This, combined with the relatively low affinity of the elicited Abs, rapidly raised population-level immune pressure on these subdominant epitopes (fig. 6 ❷❸). This presumably expedited the emergence of an evolving series of highly escapable variants that independently incorporated a limited subset of divergent S-associated mutations that converged to more conserved sites within S-RBD and/or S-NTD. Most recent immune escape variants were selected on the basis of their incorporation of variant-specific infection-enhancing mutations that converged to S-RBD and thereby evaded the infection-inhibiting Ab response elicited in previously mRNA-vaccinated individuals (or presumably also in vaccinated individuals who experienced PNNAb-dependent VBTIs) (ref. 29). As these newly emerged highly infectious Omicron descendants do not induce SIR-enabling VBTIs, they are not readily escapable. They cause the population to gradually increase PNNAb-mediated immune pressure on viral trans infectiousness (fig. 6 ❹).

It follows that mRNA vaccination triggered broadly neutralizing and infection-inhibiting Abs that only provided short-lived protection from disease and productive infection[53], respectively, and rapidly paved the way to the co-emergence/co-circulation of highly infectious Omicron descendants. It is therefore fair to conclude that mRNA vaccines–akin to SIR-enabling VBTIs–could at most enable the host immune system to temporarily delay the immune escape dynamics of the virus to then expedite those dynamics by triggering large-scale immune escape.

Updated mRNA booster doses (i.e., comprising Omicron-adapted S-encoding mRNA) administered before highly infectious Omicron descendants co-emerged likely triggered SIR 2 upon exposure of vaccinated individuals to newly emerged Omicron-derived variants (fig. 3). By triggering a SIR event, alone or in combination with productive infection, they likely further promoted viral immune escape.

However, even if administered after the highly infectious Omicron descendant emerged, updated/Omicron-adapted booster doses would only expedite immune escape dynamics. Due to their high intrinsic infectiousness, these co-circulating lineages provoke *Ab-independent* VBTIs in the vaccinated. While the latter do not provoke SIR, they enhance uptake of highly infectious progeny virions into APCs and thereby prevent priming of new Abs by vaccinal Ags (chapters 7.2. and 8.2.). On the other hand, the Omicron-adapted Ag would not result in recall of previously vaccine-primed Abs due to the important antigenic differences between the S Ag of recently emerged Omicron descendants and the S antigen used in the original vaccine (i.e., derived from Wuhan-Hu lineage). In other words, updated Omicron booster doses will be unable to abolish or even delay the gradually growing PNNAb-mediate immune pressure that highly vaccinated populations are currently placing on viral virulence (chapter 1.2.10.). The increase in this immune pressure is now solely determined by the scale and frequency of *Ab-independent* VBTIs in highly vaccinated populations. PNNAb-independent VBTIs are therefore driving the emergence of virulence-enhancing immune escape mutations.

Chapter Eight

The more you train (the CBIIS), the more you gain; the more you vaccinate (during a pandemic), the more you deteriorate (the adaptive immune response).

8.1. Natural infection but not vaccination trains the CBIIS and therefore avoids SIR-enabling, PNNAb-dependent BTI and prevents viral immune escape. mRNA vaccination, however, promotes SIR and therefore abrogates cell-based innate immune training while promoting PNNAb-mediated VBTIs and therefore expedites immune escape.

*Mass immunization during a natural pandemic (of a virus causing acute self-limiting infection) not only generates herd immunity but also provides long-lived protection to the individual while preventing immune_escape. In contrast, **mass immunization through mass vaccination** during a pandemic drives viral immune_escape and generates immune escape variants (e.g., OOV/EOSVs) that provoke large-scale SIR-enabling VBTIs. Although the latter provide some short-lived immune protection, they compromise CBII training and dramatically expedite large-scale immune escape. The latter generates highly infectious immune escape variants that are currently generating increasing herd immune pressure on viral virulence.*

The statement above is supported by an immunological rationale and in-depth molecular and biological analysis of evolving variants (as compared to data from literature on viral lineages that circulated during the <u>natural</u> influenza pandemic of 1918 (refs. 11 and 12). It also relies on reports summarizing clinical observations made during the current pandemic. In this book, I am not discussing these reports/publications in detail, but have rather used their overall findings to fine-tune my hypothesis and to validate the proposed immunological mechanism and my predictions. A non-exhaustive list of the publications I consulted can be found under 'consulted literature' at the end of this book (with special emphasis on refs. 13-32).

Clinical observations made during the current pandemic have, for example, shown that the protective effect against infection conferred by natural priming of children during the pandemic was much more prolonged compared to the protection conferred following regular mRNA vaccination in infection-primed or unprimed children (ref. 45: see fig. 1, graphs C and B, respectively).

Graph C shows how during the pre-Delta phase of the pandemic, primary infection conferred prolonged protection against reinfection by subsequent variants.

Natural immunity not only conferred prolonged protection against productive infection but also mitigated disease symptoms and hospitalization rates (as reflected by comparing graph F as compared to graph E (ref. 45: see fig.1).

Even though NBTIs may occasionally have occurred in unvaccinated individuals,[54] it is reasonable to assume that the frequency thereof during the pre-Omicron phase of the pandemic was much lower than that of VBTIs in mRNA-vaccinated individuals, regardless of previous infection. This can be concluded from the steeper decline in immune protection/responses depicted in graphs D and B compared to graph C (ref. 45: see fig.1).

The observation that mRNA-based vaccination[55] during the pandemic only provided short-lived protection against Omicron descendants and further declined upon emergence of EOSVs is entirely in line with the postulate that mRNA vaccination triggers SIR (fig. 5 panel D). In addition, there is now ample evidence from the literature that VBTIs are associated with rapid changes in the spectrum and characteristics of anti-S Abs in highly vaccinated populations (refs. 21-23 and 25-27). All the above strongly suggests that SIR-enabling vaccines (i.e., mRNA-based vaccines) critically contributed to the rapidly evolving sequence of new emerging variants.

Based upon the comparison between the effectiveness of previous pre-Delta, Delta and Omicron infection against reinfection (as a function of time since previous infection), it can be concluded that the longevity of natural immune protection against reinfection declined with a higher level of infectiousness[56] of the new emerging variant (in comparison to the priming lineage) (ref. 45: see fig. 1, graph C). The similarly rapid decline in protection against infection with Omicron in the unvaccinated and the vaccinated seems to indicate that both subpopulations experienced BTIs following exposure to Omicron (the decline shown for Omicron in graphs C and D is steep and very similar). Given the enhanced infection rate caused by dominant circulation of more infectious pre-Omicron variants, it is indeed reasonable to assume that BTIs have regularly occurred in the unvaccinated, however without triggering SIR (chapters 3.8., 6.1. and 6.2.).

Although the co-circulating newly emerged Omicron descendants are highly infectious due to the incorporation of infection-enhancing motifs in their S-RBD, continuous training of the CBIIS (via exposure) has enabled the unvaccinated to successfully adapt their first line of immune defense to a more infectious environment and to eliminate most of the viral load at an early stage of infection. This explains why the majority of unvaccinated individuals experienced at most some <u>mild</u> disease symptoms upon exposure to these highly infectious lineages. This is in sharp contrast to the situation in vaccinated individuals who do not control virus infection at all and are now experiencing more and more Ab-independent VBTIs.

Interestingly enough, the clinical outcome (in terms of symptoms) for the unvaccinated and vaccinated is now quite comparable, although the immune protective mechanisms involved are fundamentally different. Whereas enhanced sterilizing immune capacity of the CBIIS improved protection against productive infection in the unvaccinated, enhanced PNNAb-mediated inhibition of viral *trans* infectiousness and activation of MHC-unrestricted CTLs is now protecting vaccinated individuals against (severe) disease.

It should also be noted that individuals who experienced asymptomatic/mild infection and did not receive more than 2 post-infection injections with a non-mRNA-based vaccine may still manage to avoid SIR-enabling VBTIs (fig. 1). However, this does not apply to individuals who received mRNA vaccines. This is because mRNA-based vaccines are likely to trigger SIR when administered after productive SC-infection, even if the latter is mild/asymptomatic (fig.1) (chapters 1.2.1. and 1.2.2.).

8.2. Why are updated mRNA booster shots (including bivalent vaccines) completely worthless?

Both wild-type spike protein of SC-2 (which is present in the original vaccines) and S protein of the Omicron BA.1 and BA. 4-5 subvariants (Moderna and Pfizer BioNTech) promote SIR by inducing low affinity Abs to S protein that mask the immunodominant S-associated epitopes expressed on the surface of free circulating S protein released from mRNA-transfected host cells. However, SIR-enabling mRNA-based booster doses can at most restimulate previously primed low-affinity memory B cells in vaccinated individuals (i.e., as a result of previous mRNA-based vaccination or SIR-enabling VBTIs). However, these pNAbs no longer work against the currently co-circulating Omicron descendants. In addition, Ab-dependent VBTIs provoked by these highly infectious variants do not allow for *de novo* priming of new Abs.

The question therefore arises as to whether updated, so-called 'Omicron-adapted' booster doses could trigger *de novo* priming of variant S-specific Abs in vaccinated individuals who are exposed to these highly infectious variants. However, as Ab-independent VBTIs in vaccinated individuals promote enhanced viral uptake into APCs, any vaccinal Ag will be outcompeted by highly infectious progeny virus for uptake into APCs[57]. This will prevent updated vaccine booster doses from priming new Abs that match the updated vaccinal S variant. In other words, the current landscape in highly vaccinated countries is now fully dominated by Ab-independent VBTIs that are largely protective against symptoms and largely accompanied by negative RT-PCR test results (as viral shedding is largely controlled by enhanced CTL activity).

On the other hand, administration of updated mRNA vaccines to previously *unvaccinated* individuals could either result in lack of vaccine 'take' (due to neutralization of the updated vaccinal S Ag by matching pre-existing anti-Omicron Abs elicited upon previous natural infection) or generate new, 'updated' Abs against the highly infectious, co-circulating Omicron descendants. However, due to the high intrinsic infectiousness of these newly emerged variants, the new neutralizing Abs would only interact with the virus after an Ab-independent VBTI has taken place. These VBTIs will only occur in unvaccinated individuals lacking a properly trained CBIIS. In this case, highly infectious progeny virus is likely to readily attach in high concentration to migratory DCs. As a result, only a minority of progeny virions would not adsorb onto DCs and be neutralized by the matching pre-existing NAbs. This would however leave unvaccinated individuals with an untrained or insufficiently trained CBIIS highly susceptible to contracting severe disease.

In conclusion, once highly infectious Omicron descendants are circulating, Ab-independent VBTIs monopolize the scene and gradually increase PNNAb-mediated immune pressure on viral virulence in highly vaccinated countries. Updated vaccine booster doses cannot change or even mitigate this situation as they both fail to prime functional Abs and do not allow recall of vaccine-primed Abs. Even in unvaccinated individuals whose immune system lacks previous training and who are therefore unprotected against severe disease upon exposure to highly infectious variants, updated Omicron-adapted vaccines would not provide added benefit.

8.3. By sidelining the CBIIS and catalyzing large-scale immune escape, PNNAb-dependent VBTIs enabled co-emergence of highly infectious Omicron descendants that are now causing highly vaccinated populations to place growing immune pressure on viral *trans* infectiousness. This is a recipe for a catastrophe.

PNNAb-dependent VBTIs enable SIR and thereby sideline the CBIIS (i.e., SIR-1 and SIR-2 in figs. 4 and 7). It is therefore fair to state that PNNAb-dependent VBTIs caused viral immune escape from both the *innate cell-mediated* and *the humoral adaptive immune system*. Immune escape from the CBIIS results in a higher susceptibility to productive infection whereas immune escape from the humoral adaptive immune system promotes co-circulation of highly infectious immune escape variants and therefore fosters growth of PNNAb-mediated immune pressure on viral *trans* infectiousness/virulence.

To abolish this population-level immune pressure the virus will need to evolve a variant that is able to release the emergency brake in use by the majority of the vaccinated to prevent severe disease. Viral escape from PNNAb-dependent inhibition of viral *trans* infection is therefore likely to independently select new, more virulent variants that will likely be streamlined into a single dominant variant. The latter will unleash its high virulence once it experiences sufficient population-level immune pressure. I predict that such a fully NAb-resistant, highly virulent variant (i.e., HIVICRON) will cause asynchronous waves of AIESD in highly vaccinated populations.

THE INESCAPABLE IMMUNE ESCAPE PANDEMIC

8.4. Individuals who only received a primary series of non-mRNA-based vaccines and did not develop clinically relevant symptoms during the pre-Omicron phase of the pandemic most likely avoided SIR-enabling VBTIs upon subsequent exposure to Omicron (sub)variants. They may therefore continue maintenance training of their CBIIS. How do we distinguish vaccinated individuals who preserved their CBIIS training capacity from those who didn't?

Widespread resistance of Omicron to Wuhan Hu-specific vaccine-induced pNAbs has ultimately led to a high incidence of PNNAb-mediated VBTIs in highly vaccinated populations; this evolution allowed the virus to sideline the CBIIS while enabling recalled memory Th cells to prime new humoral immune responses to more conserved, subdominant epitopes. By triggering SIR and thus promoting large-scale immune escape, *widespread* PNNAb-mediated VBTIs drove SC-2 to evolve highly infectious variants in highly vaccinated populations. These highly infectious variants are now provoking Ab-independent VBTIs in vaccinated individuals who failed to train their CBIIS with pre-Omicron variants or whose training was abrogated as a result of a SIR event.

Since failure to train or maintain the sterilizing capacity of their CBIIS puts vaccinated individuals at high risk of contracting AIESD upon exposure to a highly virulent variant, it is critical from a prognostic perspective to evaluate whether or not a vaccinated person has managed to align training of the CBIIS to the growing level of infectiousness of circulating variants.

Symptomatic infection that occurred in vaccinated individuals during the pre-Omicron phase of the pandemic could not be due to PNNAb-dependent VBTIs as the neutralizing capacity of previously primed pNAbs towards pre-Omicron variants was not low enough to elicit PNNAbs. One can, therefore, conclude that PNNAb-dependent VBTIs did not occur during the pre-Omicron phase and therefore, symptomatic infection during the pre-Omicron phase did not bypass the CBIIS.

However, if first symptoms of disease in vaccinated individuals were only acquired after the advent of Omicron, it is impossible to know whether or not the PNNAb-dependent BTIs that provoked disease triggered SIR and hence, whether they had sidelined the CBIIS. 'Trained' vaccinated individuals who contracted a PNNAb-dependent BTI that failed to trigger SIR developed non-severe symptoms of disease to the same extent as unvaccinated individuals who experienced a PNNAb-dependent NBTI upon exposure to OOV or EOSVs shortly after their previous productive infection with a pre-Omicron variant) (fig. 5 panel A and fig. 7). On the other hand, vaccinated individuals who contracted SIR-enabling PNNAb-dependent VBTIs could equally contract disease while being protected from severe symptoms[58] after having experienced a limited episode (presumably 1-3 months) of protection against productive infection [59].

However, even in the current stage of the pandemic (characterized by co-circulation of highly infectious Omicron descendants), it is still impossible to clinically distinguish between vaccinated individuals who preserved maintenance training of their CBIIS and those who didn't. Vaccinated individuals who preserved their CBII maintenance training and were exposed to a highly infectious variant shortly after previous exposure to OOV or EOSV may still have developed PNNAb-mediated BTIs while being protected from severe disease (due to PNNAb-mediated inhibition of viral *trans* infectiousness/virulence). However, their susceptibility to PNNAb-mediated BTIs (and hence, to disease altogether) is likely to gradually decrease as a consequence of diminished shedding of the co-circulating highly infectious variants (chapters 3.2., 3.3. and 6.2.) and reduced infectiousness of more virulent Omicron descendants (ref. 57). On the other hand, vaccinated individuals whose CBII maintenance training was prevented or abrogated because of a SIR-enabling event are now subject to Ab-independent VBTIs. As the latter sustain PNNAb-mediated inhibition of viral *trans* infectiousness/virulence while enhancing activation of CTL-mediated viral clearance (chapter 4.2.), vaccinated individuals who did not preserve sufficient training capacity of their CBIIS are equally well protected from severe disease while gradually decreasing their susceptibility to disease altogether.

Based on the above, it is not possible to use clinical data or medical histories to assess whether or not a vaccinated individual who contracted symptomatic infection during the Omicron phase of the pandemic and subsequently refrained from mRNA vaccination still had/has the capacity to train the CBIIS.

Unfortunately, there are currently no validated assays that can directly assess the level of innate cell-based immune training. However, it is possible to infer from the individual's pre-symptomatic vaccine history whether capability to train the CBIIS has been preserved.

Failure to train the CBIIS likely occurred when unvaccinated individuals received 3 doses of a non-mRNA-based vaccine or 2 doses of an mRNA-based vaccine, at least one of which was mRNA-based, prior to contracting symptomatic infection. Failure to continue training of the CBIIS likely occurred when unvaccinated individuals who experienced symptomatic infection during the pre-Omicron phase of the pandemic subsequently received one dose of a vaccine. In the case of mRNA-based vaccines, a single injection even after an *asymptomatic/mild* infection would suffice to trigger SIR (fig. 1).

On the other hand, vaccinated individuals who do not fall into these categories likely avoided SIR-mediating VBTIs and were therefore able to preserve maintenance training of their CBIIS upon exposure to pre-Omicron and/or Omicron(-derived) lineages. This would typically apply to vaccinated individuals who only received one vaccine shot, or at most 2 vaccine shots with a non-mRNA-based vaccine, before they contracted symptomatic infection or who received one or 2 doses of a non-mRNA-based vaccine after having experienced an asymptomatic/mild infection.

8.5. Viral exposure to OOV or EOSV after priming with mRNA vaccines or after boosting with non-mRNA vaccines triggered SIR. As SIR prevented training of the CBIIS, many vaccinated individuals now solely depend on PNNAbs for controlling severe disease.

SIR-enabling VBTIs or SIR-enabling vaccination (i.e., mRNA-based vaccination) sidelines the CBIIS and redirects the humoral immune response at (subdominant) S protein-associated epitopes expressed on the surface of free-circulating virion or S protein (the latter in the case of mRNA vaccination). SIR prevents or abrogates training of the CBIIS and drives viral immune escape. SIR therefore expedited the occurrence of widespread PNNAb-mediated VBTIs in highly vaccinated populations (fig. 4). This entailed irrevocable sidelining of the CBIIS. Vaccinated individuals who experienced SIR have been subject to PNNAb-dependent VBTIs for as long as they were not exposed to new, highly infectious immune escape variants, the emergence of which resulted from SIR-mediated immune escape. Highly infectious immune escape variants trigger (PNN)Ab-independent VBTIs and thereby enable vaccinated individuals to control severe disease via PNNAb-mediated inhibition of viral *trans* infectiousness.

I am inferring this from my immunological understanding that previous infection-primed immunity could enable SIR, and thus abrogate training of the CBIIS, upon subsequent vaccination (fig. 1). But even vaccination in previously *uninfected* individuals can trigger SIR. This is, for example, the case when productive infection (or administration of an *mRNA* booster dose) occurs after administration of a primary series of an *mRNA* vaccine. In previously uninfected individuals who received non-mRNA vaccines, SIR could only be triggered in case the vaccinated individual contracted a PNNAb-dependent VBTI (fig. 7). PNNAb-dependent VBTIs occur upon exposure of vaccine-boosted individuals to OOV or EOSVs.

As SIR-enabling vaccines or VBTIs prevent training of the CBIIS, the vast majority of vaccinated individuals are bound to rely on PNNAbs to control severe disease. Whereas both trained CBII and virulence-neutralizing PNNAbs are variant-nonspecific, trained CBII is endowed with immunological memory while B cells producing Th-independent PNNAbs have no memory.

In other words, protection of many vaccinated individuals is now fully dependent on the virulence-neutralizing PNNAbs, the activity of which can only be sustained provided their production is continuously stimulated. However, the production of PNNAbs is currently compromised by repeated viral exposure and declining vaccinal Ab titers (chapter 3.1.).

Chapter Nine

Mass Vaccination: From NAb-dependent protection against disease to Ab-independent enhancement of severe disease. (figs. 2, 8 and 9)

The diminished neutralizability of dominantly circulating Omicron has undeniably resulted from mass vaccination during the pandemic. Omicron's diminished neutralizability has rapidly been followed by large-scale SIR-enabling VBTIs in highly vaccinated populations. Taken together, it is fair to conclude that the escalation of immune escape variants witnessed since the advent of Omicron is indirectly rooted in the mass vaccination program. Because Omicron massively caused SIR-enabling VBTIs in highly vaccinated populations, it has prevented the untrained CBIIS of vaccinated individuals from effectively controlling infection of currently co-circulating, highly infectious variants which fulminant SIR-mediated immune escape eventually generated.

In conclusion, it is reasonable to state that in highly vaccinated populations, Omicron managed to self-catalyze its evolution into highly infectious descendants and thereby paved the way to the likely emergence of new, more virulent immune escape variants that will ultimately culminate in natural selection of HIVICRON, which will likely be characterized by a combination of enhanced intrinsic infectiousness, NAb-evasiveness and high virulence. One can therefore only conclude that Omicron has been anything but a blessing and that the scourge it presents is to be entirely blamed on the mass vaccination program.

Pre-omicron variants were characterized by a diversified spectrum of evolving mutations that converged to the variant-specific RBD. The resulting antigenic drift in mutational hotspots progressively conferred increased resistance to a diversified spectrum of more variant-specific functional Abs. Those progressively evolved their activity from predominantly infection-inhibiting to predominantly virus-neutralizing. In response to the rising population-level immune pressure the virus eventually evolved into Omicron. Omicron enabled a spectacular expansion of viral immune-evasive capacity. This is because Omicron triggered widespread PNNAb-dependent VBTIs in highly vaccinated populations and thereby rapidly enabled the population to place high immune pressure on more conserved, neutralizing and infection-facilitating domains of S protein (via SIR). This required EOSVs to rapidly escape from broadly functional Abs (i.e., by successively incorporating a limited subset of shared, highly variant-specific mutations in conserved regions of NTD and RBD[60]). Large-scale immune escape eventually drove co-circulation of highly infectious Omicron descendants that are now triggering Ab-independent VBTIs that cause highly vaccinated populations to place gradually increasing immune pressure on viral virulence.

While our experts cheered on the exciting potential of mRNA vaccinations/boosters and VBTIs to induce broadly cross-functional Abs that could even protect against productive infection and would always protect against severe disease, they seem to have ignored that both prevented training of the CBIIS and triggered large scale immune escape. By curtailing the capacity of the CBIIS to train, VBTIs with Omicron have forced vaccinated individuals to exclusively put their protection in the hands of vaccinal Abs, which–since the advent of Omicron–have directly or indirectly (i.e., via SIR) expedited large-scale immune escape. Consequently, the landscape became rapidly dominated by co-circulating highly infectious variants which are now responsible for a gradual, large-scale increase in population-level immunity on viral virulence. It therefore appears highly likely that Ab-independent enhancement of intrinsic viral infectiousness of co-circulating variants will soon evolve into Ab-independent enhancement of intrinsic viral virulence and hence, propulse a wave of AIESD in highly vaccinated countries/regions.

Based on the above, one can reasonably conclude that with the advent of Omicron in highly vaccinated populations, viral immune escape dynamics triggered by the mass vaccination program had reached a point of no return. The reason for this disastrous evolution must be sought in SIR, which allowed OOV and derived immune escape variants to self-catalyze and expedite large-scale immune escape. As the latter is currently driven by co-circulating, highly infectious variants, each highly vaccinated country/region should be considered in the process of selecting an immune escape variant endowed with high virulence potential.

Because PNNAbs bind to a conserved antigenic site within S-NTD, OOV and all EOSVs that can no longer be sufficiently neutralized by pre-existing pNAbs acquired enhanced infectiousness (i.e., via binding of said conserved antigenic site to the same PNNAbs) in vaccinated individuals. Likewise, all highly infectious Omicron [sub]variants that can no longer be sufficiently inhibited by pre-existing virulence-neutralizing Abs acquire enhanced virulence (i.e., by preventing said conserved antigenic site from binding to the same PNNAbs). Hindrance of PNNAb binding presumably occurs via O-glycosite mutations (ref. 5) and) causing Ab-independent enhancement of severe disease.

I have no doubt that the advent of Omicron will be remembered in the history of mankind as a pivotal moment. Mass vaccination turned a natural viral pandemic into a viral *immune escape pandemic*, and Omicron turned the immune escape pandemic into an *inescapable* immune escape pandemic (fig. 12). This means that in highly vaccinated countries, Omicron irreversibly and irrevocably forced the immune escape pandemic into an evolution that can no longer be halted by large-scale host immunity–it will only be halted by large-scale decimation of the host population. This will go down in history as the most devastating but unambiguous example of how Nature mercilessly punishes man's incredibly naive belief that through technology, he can control biology.

Chapter Ten

Conclusions

The key difference between natural infection and vaccination is that natural infection trains the CBIIS while vaccination (using non-replicating vaccines) does not. The latter is particularly problematic when mass vaccination programs are conducted during a pandemic (of a virus causing acute self-limiting infection) as Abs will take time to mature (i.e., to acquire full affinity and functionality). Large scale induction of low-affinity Abs to S protein during a pandemic initially places suboptimal population-level immune pressure on viral infectiousness and subsequently (i.e., as vaccine-induced NAbs mature) on viral neutralizability; this eventually promotes natural selection and dominant propagation of more infectious and less neutralizable variants. However, during the pre-Omicron phase of this immune escape pandemic, high titers of high-affinity NAbs protected vaccinated individuals against disease, and people with a weak CBIIS (e.g., due to comorbidities, advanced age or underlying immune compromising conditions) therefore benefitted from vaccination. In contrast, unvaccinated immunologically naïve people had to fully rely on their CBIIS to fight off SC-2. Many of them–with the exception of young children and other healthy individuals with strong CBII–contracted mostly moderate disease symptoms upon their first exposure to the virus. The unvaccinated elderly or those unvaccinated with co-morbidities regularly progressed to developing severe disease.

However, once unvaccinated healthy subjects had experienced productive infection, their CBIIS developed adaptive memory, which is the optimal immune defense for anyone caught in an *immune escape pandemic.* This is because functional reprogramming of imprinted innate immune cells (i.e., NK cells) allows for elimination of SC-2-infected cells at an early stage of viral infection, regardless of the variant. As a 'trained' CBIIS will eliminate the bulk of viral load shortly after the onset of the infection, healthy, infection-experienced unvaccinated individuals become less susceptible to productive infection and disease upon re-exposure. Even in the case of more infectious variants, a properly trained CBIIS will confer improved protection against disease[61] and NBTI. As the

CBIIS diminishes the viral load, NBTIs will not give rise to SIR and therefore not promote immune escape.

Though the virus has been continuously upgrading its infectious behavior (as a consequence of population-level immune pressure), the vast majority of vaccinated individuals have no choice but to rely upon their vaccinal Abs (as vaccines are non-replicating and therefore do not allow training of the CBIIS, often preventing or abrogating CBIIS training). Highly vaccinated countries witnessed massive cases of PNNAb-dependent VBTIs when the neutralizing capacity of vaccine-induced Abs dramatically decreased as a result of spectacular viral immune escape (i.e., due to Omicron). After a short episode of enhanced immune protection, large-scale SIR-enabling VBTIs–oftentimes fueled by mRNA vaccines–broadened and increased immune pressure on viral infectiousness in highly vaccinated populations. Such large-scale PNNAb-dependent BTIs in vaccinated individuals have been instrumental in expediting large-scale viral immune escape and responsible for current co-circulation of highly infectious Omicron descendants. These new emerging variants are now triggering Ab-independent VBTIs that allow those vaccinated individuals whose CBII training was prevented or abrogated to gradually raise immune pressure on viral virulence while experiencing mitigated disease symptoms. In contrast, mitigation of disease symptoms in the unvaccinated occurs through enhanced elimination of these highly infectious immune escape variants via their trained CBIIS.

Selectional adaptation of viral immune escape variants to large-scale enhanced immune pressure on viral *trans* infectiousness/virulence is likely to select a new type of SC-variant fully capable of breaking through vaccine-mediated immune protection against severe disease and thereby enabling the virus to spread and replicate in different distal organs of vaccinated individuals. I predict that such Ab-independent enhancement of severe disease (AIESD) will exclusively occur in vaccinated individuals who did not develop sufficient cell-based innate immune capacity. In contrast, maintenance training of their CBIIS as a result of continued exposure to newly emerging variants will protect the healthy unvaccinated from AIESD and even from disease altogether.

With this understanding, it is fair to postulate that by provoking SIR-enabling VBTIs, viral immune escape from variant S-specific pNAbs[62] has a self-catalyzing effect that expedites the co-emergence of highly infectious immune escape variants. The latter cause highly vaccinated populations to gradually place growing population-level immune pressure on viral virulence while temporarily improving protection of vaccinated individuals against disease.

I cannot imagine how the majority of vaccinated individuals in highly vaccinated countries (especially in countries predominantly using mRNA-based vaccines) would not succumb to viral variants adaptively evolved to abolish the increasing, large-scale immune pressure these very vaccinated individuals are currently exerting on viral virulence. As the mass vaccination program is undoubtedly at the origin of this evolution, it must be considered the largest and most dangerous *in vivo* gain-of-function experiment ever conducted in the history of biology– *one which mankind has unleashed on its very own species.*

It is highly likely that mass immunization with mRNA vaccine technology only served to expedite the above-described evolutionary path of the virus in highly vaccinated populations. It is also highly likely that those who received mRNA-based vaccines will be particularly at risk of contracting AIESD, as many of them are unlikely to have preserved sufficient cell-based innate immune capacity. This is because mRNA vaccines trigger SIR even in the absence of infection, and can also abrogate training of the CBIIS in those who previously experienced asymptomatic/mild infection. Based on immunological considerations, it is reasonable to assume that any mRNA-based vaccination performed after infection, or any productive infection or S protein-based mRNA booster dose (updated or otherwise) in previously mRNA vaccine-primed individuals triggered immune refocusing; this would have also prevented or even abrogated training of innate immune cells.

It is therefore highly likely that large-scale administration of mRNA-based vaccines/booster doses rapidly increased the level and breadth of population-level immune pressure on viral infectiousness and ultimately on viral *trans* infectiousness. One can reasonably postulate that usage of mRNA vaccine technology in this mass vaccination program expedited large-scale immune escape and will only precipitate a catastrophic wave of mortality in highly vaccinated populations.

I have always speculated that in order for the virus to resist to PNNAb-mediated suppression of viral virulence (which is now critical for the virus to survive given its diminished transmissibility), selected mutations would need to involve changes in the O-glycosylation profile of S protein in ways that lift the PNNAb blockade on viral *trans* infectiousness/virulence (ref. 5). However, the impact of such O-glycosite mutations would only come to fruition if (productive) infection by currently circulating, highly infectious variants cannot be controlled by the CBIIS. I therefore predict that all healthy unvaccinated individuals who've trained their CBIIS during this immune escape pandemic will be protected from severe disease and even from the disease altogether. The combination of high susceptibility to AIESD in vaccinated individuals and strong sterilizing CBII in the healthy unvaccinated is likely to eradicate the highly infectious Omicron descendants in highly vaccinated regions and thereby end the immune escape pandemic.

In summary, PNNAb-mediating VBTIs are to be considered the key mechanism by which OOV, a dominantly circulating variant with diminished sensitivity to a multitude of pre-Omicron lineage-specific neutralizing Abs, irreversibly self-catalyzed viral immune escape dynamics. Expedited viral immune escape eventually resulted in co-circulation of several highly infectious Omicron descendants now causing highly vaccinated populations to exert gradually growing, widespread immune pressure on viral virulence. This evolution is likely to culminate in natural selection of a new type of variant ('HIVICRON') that has the capacity to rapidly and massively trigger AIESD in vaccinated individuals. In contrast, healthy unvaccinated individuals with continued exposure during this immune escape pandemic will be unaffected. I can only conclude that the threat of a tsunami suddenly disrupting the calmness of the current landscape is now imminent in highly vaccinated populations.

Chapter Eleven

Answers To Key Questions

11.1. Why and how did VBTIs with Omicron self-catalyze immune escape?

While having provided some initial short-lived protection against productive infection (and hence, against viral immune escape), VBTIs with Omicron expedited viral immune escape from NAbs and gave rise to new Omicron descendants that are now paving the way to viral immune escape from PNNAbs.

VBTIs with Omicron triggered SIR-1. Immune masking[63] by Abs that mismatch the immunodominant S-associated target epitopes prevented the latter from recalling their corresponding neutralizing Abs while enabling previously outcompeted[64], more conserved subdominant S-associated epitopes to prime broadly neutralizing Abs of weak affinity that only provide short-lived protection. By placing high immune pressure on their corresponding conserved epitopes, these low-affinity Abs rapidly promoted natural immune selection and co-circulation of Omicron variants that could escape from these broadly neutralizing Abs. By incorporating a limited subset of shared mutations specific to the ancestral Wuhan-Hu lineage into more conserved S-associated domains, these variants rendered the targeted S-associated domains less recognizable by the broadly NAbs.

Upon subsequent PNNAb-dependent VBTIs with these new immune escape variants, pre-existing vaccine- and SIR-primed pNAbs likely bound to the S-associated immunodominant and mutated epitopes, respectively; this presumably triggered SIR-2 and caused *de novo* priming of new Abs of low affinity that were directed at more conserved S-associated domains that facilitate viral infection. By placing high immune pressure on their corresponding conserved epitopes, these low-affinity Abs promoted natural immune selection and co-circulation of Omicron variants that could escape from these broadly infection-inhibiting Abs by incorporating a subset of shared mutations that mediated enhanced viral infectiousness of specific pre-Omicron variants (i.e., Beta, Gamma, Delta variant).

Because SIR-1 and SIR-2 allowed a subset of subdominant S-associated epitopes to prime entirely new B cells, the S protein selected to adorn the currently co-circulating highly infectious Omicron-derived immune escape (sub)variants is very different from the previous variants (i.e., BA.2-derived variants such as Omicron BA.4/5, XBB and BQ.1.1. variants as compared to OOV). These co-circulating, highly infectious Omicron descendants are now causing widespread Ab-independent VBTIs and thereby cause highly vaccinated populations to place PNNAb-mediated immune pressure viral *trans* infectiousness/virulence.

THE INESCAPABLE IMMUNE ESCAPE PANDEMIC

11.2. How did 'original antigenic sin' and SIR contribute to viral immune escape?

In highly vaccinated populations, exposure to pre-Omicron variants has caused viral immune escape from variant S-specific neutralizing Abs through 'antigenic sin', whereas exposure to Omicron (sub)variants has triggered viral immune escape from variant S-nonspecific infection-inhibiting Abs through SIR.

It is fair to state that the phenomenon of 'original antigenic sin' and that of 'steric immune refocusing' exacerbated the dramatic effect of intra-pandemic mass vaccination on immune escape in the pre-Omicron and Omicron phase, respectively. Whereas mass vaccination combined with re-exposure (and hence, recall of anti-S Abs) during the pre-Omicron phase drove SC-2 to escape from variant S-specific neutralizing Abs, SIR-enabling VBTIs during the Omicron phase have been driving SC-2 to evolve new variants capable of escaping from broadly functional Abs. While natural immune selection of a single variant (i.e., OOV) following mass vaccination during a pandemic allowed SC-2 to immediately escape from variant S-specific Nabs in the majority of vaccinated individuals, natural immune selection of a diversified set of highly infectious Omicron-derived subvariants following SIR-enabling VBTIs allowed SC-2 to rapidly escape from variant-nonspecific infection-inhibiting Abs. This has triggered *Ab-independent* VBTIs that are now driving immune escape from virulence-inhibiting PNNAbs and will likely result in a high incidence of *Ab-independent* enhancement of virulence/severe disease in highly vaccinated countries.

11.3. Why is maintenance training of the CBIIS a blessing?

A trained CBIIS diminishes viral load at an early stage of infection and thereby prevents SIR, even in the case of PNNAb-dependent NBTIs. In the absence of SIR, the CBIIS maintains its capacity to adapt its sterilizing immune capacity to the higher infectiousness of circulating immune escape variants ('immune escape pandemic'). Trained CBII therefore improves the individual's protection against disease while reducing viral transmission in the population (which is key to establish herd immunity).

11.4. Why is mass vaccination during the pandemic a scourge and particularly problematic when mRNA-based vaccines are used?

This is because non-replicating C-19 vaccines are directed at a protein (i.e., S protein) that is responsible for viral infectiousness. Mass vaccination during a natural SC-2 pandemic drives natural selection of more infectious viruses and eventually results in population-level immune pressure on viral virulence (fig. 6). mRNA-based vaccination in particular expedites the occurrence of PNNAb-dependent, SIR-enabling VBTIs in vaccinated individuals while preventing or abrogating CBIIS training.

Upon first exposure to a pre-Omicron variant, the CBIIS of an unvaccinated healthy individual removed a substantial amount of the viral load at an early stage of infection; less virus was therefore taken up by tissue-resident APCs. This resulted in relatively low and short-lived anti-S Ab titers (in comparison to vaccine-induced Ab titers) and therefore reduced the risk for an unvaccinated to contract PNNAb-dependent NBTI upon subsequent exposure to OOV or EOSVs (fig. 5: panel B).

Prior training of the CBIIS as facilitated by pre-Omicron lineages (including the ancestral Wuhan-Hu strain) substantially slowed down the production rate of progeny virus in the case the unvaccinated experienced PNNAb-dependent NBTI with Omicron. The latter can occur upon exposure at a time when pNAb titers from previous infection (i.e., with a pre-Omicron variant) have not yet sufficiently waned. However, because a trained CBIIS of a healthy person will reduce the production rate of progeny virus, pre-existing S-specific pNAbs will bind in relatively higher concentration to the released progeny virions. Binding of pNAbs in sufficiently high concentration to progeny virus would enable fast and abundant viral uptake into APCs, thereby preventing SIR and promoting cytolytic destruction of virus-infected cells by activated CTL. PNNAb-dependent NBTIs therefore do not compromise training of the CBIIS and also prevent SC-2 from driving immune escape while enabling a swift recovery from disease (fig. 5 panel A and fig. 7).

In contrast, vaccination tends to elicit high and long-lived pNAb titers without concomitant training of the CBIIS. Long-lived elevated pNAb titers combined with untrained or insufficiently trained CBII explain why PNNAb-dependent VBTIs with Omicron occur much more frequently than PNNAb-dependent NBTIs in highly vaccinated populations. It also explains why the former triggers SIR during infection with Omicron (fig. 5 panel C and fig. 7).

The combination of elevated titers of pre-existing pNAbs along with the absence of trained CBII makes it more likely for VBTIs to enable SIR (fig 5 panel C and fig. 7). Such PNNAb-dependent VBTIs result in a high production rate of progeny virus. It is therefore reasonable to assume that pre-existing S-specific pNAbs bind in relatively lower concentration to released SC-2 progeny virions. The average circulation time of these pNAb-virus complexes is therefore thought to be prolonged and their average uptake into tissue-resident APCs (and hence, recovery from Covid-19 disease) delayed. This would leave enough time for these complexes to trigger SIR and thereby induce broadly neutralizing or infection-inhibiting Abs. The refocused functional immune response prevents training of the CBIIS and expedites viral immune escape (figs. 3, 4 and 7). Large-scale immune escape eventually leads to co-emergence/co-circulation of highly infectious Omicron descendants that drive a large number of Ab-independent BTI in vaccinated individuals. Such VBTIs are now gradually increasing widespread PNNAb-mediated immune pressure on viral virulence in highly vaccinated populations (chapter 1.2.10.).

SIR-enabling vaccinations (i.e., mRNA-based vaccination) compromise the CBIIS of vaccinated individuals while promoting the frequency and expediting the occurrence of PNNAb-dependent VBTIs. It is therefore fair to assume that mRNA-based vaccines have substantially contributed to driving immune escape and raising population-level immune pressure on viral virulence (figs. 1, 4, 5 panel D and 7) (chapters 1.2.1., 1.2.2., 7. , 7.2. and 8.2.). Because of immune refocusing (i.e., failure to neutralize EOSVs) or inability to prime new Abs (i.e., failure to neutralize late/recent Omicron-derived subvariants), even new (i.e., Omicron-updated) mRNA-based bivalent vaccines failed to improve protection in previously vaccinated individuals. However, they were still able to boost previously primed broadly neutralizing Abs that–due to their diminished neutralizing capacity towards newly emerged Omicron variants–are prone to trigger PNNAb-dependent VBTIs. There is therefore no doubt that massive deployment of these vaccines is now placing a high percentage of vaccinated individuals in highly vaccinated populations at risk of contracting AIESD.

In summary, mass vaccination with vaccines during a pandemic is a scourge because it drives immune escape and thereby diminishes the neutralizing capacity of pNAbs. This allowed Omicron to cause large-scale PNNAb-dependent VBTIs that provoked SIR. SIR is to be considered a catastrophic event both from an individual and public health viewpoint. This is because SIR irreversibly sidelines the CBIIS during an immune escape pandemic and fuels fast and large-scale immune escape in highly vaccinated populations. This evolution has likely been expedited by the administration of mRNA-based vaccines. Enhanced immune escape has now caused the emergence of multiple new Omicron descendants that exhibit a high level of intrinsic viral infectiousness. Highly infectious Omicron descendants trigger Ab-independent VBTIs and thereby gradually raise large-scale PNNAb-mediated population-level immune pressure on viral virulence in highly vaccinated populations while lowering shedding and mitigating disease symptoms in vaccinated individuals (figs. 4 and 11) (chapters 3.1., 3.2., 3.3.).

11.5. Why was the incidence rate of disease in vaccinated individuals higher than in the unvaccinated in the early days of Omicron? Why should OOV-induced BTIs that occurred in individuals previously vaccinated with mRNA-based vaccines be considered a poor prognostic sign?

As most unvaccinated had an opportunity to train their CBIIS during the pre-Omicron phase, many only suffered mild disease symptoms following infection with the original Omicron variant (OOV). However, some unvaccinated persons manifested more pronounced disease symptoms as their re-exposure resulted in NBTIs. Such NBTIs were likely due to the high infection rate in the population combined with an important level of antigenic discrepancy (in the receptor-binding domain of S protein; S-RBD) between pre-Omicron variants and OOV. It is reasonable to assume that because of the mismatch between the OOV and pre-existing infection-primed Abs[65], unvaccinated individuals who were exposed to Omicron shortly after their previous productive infection (mostly with the Delta variant) contracted disease (although not in the severe form). It is highly likely that because of the insufficient Omicron-neutralizing capacity of their pre-existing anti-S Abs, these individuals experienced PNNAb-dependent enhancement of viral infectiousness and therefore contracted disease following PNNAb-dependent NBTI (fig. 5 panels A and C and fig. 7).

In contrast, mRNA vaccination *frequently* resulted in symptomatic PNNAb-dependent BTIs upon exposure to Omicron. This is because the threshold for mRNA-based vaccines to trigger SIR is very low (chapters 1.2.1. and 1.2.2.). A single mRNA vaccine injection in a person previously exposed to a pre-Omicron variant or administration of a primary series of vaccine injections, one of which was an mRNA vaccine, to a previously uninfected person likely sufficed to predispose that person to a PNNAb-dependent VBTI upon subsequent exposure to OOV (fig. 1). In other words, the occurrence of OOV-induced BTIs in an mRNA-vaccinated person was likely due to SIR and therefore considered a poor prognostic sign.

As SIR compromises the CBIIS, symptomatic infection following exposure to Omicron would be an ominous prognostic sign in those who received an mRNA injection during the pre-Omicron phase of the pandemic. It should be noted, however, that there are a few exceptions in which the CBIIS of vaccinated individuals may have preserved its training capacity (see chapter 8.4.; fig. 1)

11.6. Why and how did Omicron enhance large-scale immune escape in highly vaccinated populations?

Based on how viral evolutionary dynamics evolve as a function of host immune pressure (fig. 6) and a plethora of recent data from the literature, it is fair to conclude that Omicron has been driving the immune system of vaccinated individuals to re-orient the immune response towards S-associated epitopes with low but broad neutralizing or infection-enhancing capacity. My insights are fully compatible with the overwhelming amount of data from the literature documenting the evolutionary dynamics of Ab-evasive mutations and the impact thereof on the biological behavior of the virus and the dynamics of the host immune response (a not-exhaustive list of supportive literature is appended at the end of the book).

As explained above, SIR-mediating VBTIs enable low affinity binding between immunodominant S-associated epitopes on free circulating virus and pre-existing, affinity-matured Abs that are directed at a heterologous antigenic variant of S protein. Steric masking of said immunodominant epitopes allows the immune system to re-orient the immune response towards more conserved, S-associated immune subdominant antigenic sites and generate broadly neutralizing anti-S Abs that take several months for affinity maturation. Due to their low affinity, these broadly neutralizing Abs exert rapidly growing immune pressure on the corresponding S-associated target epitopes and thereby drive *large-scale viral immune escape*. In highly vaccinated populations, subsequent VBTIs caused by EOSVs that evolved to escape previously elicited broadly neutralizing or broadly infection-inhibiting anti-S Abs have been driving *co-circulation* of a diversified subset of new emerging variants that share a high level of intrinsic viral infectiousness.

11.7. How did mass vaccination during the pandemic generate a dangerous *immune escape* pandemic? (figs. 6, 8 and 9)

Vaccination generates long-lived pNAb titers while failing to train the CBIIS.

The advent of Omicron substantially enhanced the prevalence of PNNAb-dependent SIR-enabling VBTIs in highly vaccinated populations–this has expedited the immune escape dynamics and irrevocably steered the pandemic into a disastrous direction.

Mass vaccination with S-directed vaccines during the pandemic resulted in suboptimal population-level immune pressure on viral infectiousness. This drove natural selection and dominant propagation of immune escape variants that vaccine-induced Abs could not sufficiently neutralize. Consequently, infection-enhancing PNNAbs came into effect and caused PNNAb-dependent enhancement of viral infectiousness, which largely prevented or abrogated adaptation and functional reprogramming (i.e., training) of innate NK cells in vaccinated individuals.

By sidelining the CBIIS and reducing viral uptake into APCs (via adsorption of relatively low concentrations of pre-existing pNAbs onto abundantly produced progeny virions), PNNAb-dependent VBTIs caused masking of S-associated immunodominant epitopes and recall of previously induced Th memory cells. SIR-enabling VBTIs therefore enabled *de novo* priming of Abs targeting more conserved, S-associated antigenic domains. As these Abs have only short-lived functional capacity and take several months to fully mature, they rapidly exerted high immune pressure on these more conserved antigenic domains and thereby precipitated large-scale emergence of new, highly infectious immune escape variants. As exposure of vaccinated individuals to highly infectious [sub]variants sustains production of PNNAbs while also improving CTL-mediated viral clearance, it is fair to conclude that these highly infectious lineages are currently keeping themselves in check.

However, given the diminishing capacity of PNNAbs to suppress *trans* infection of highly infectious Omicron descendants, viral control is inextricably linked to a gradual and widespread increase in PNNAb-mediated population-level immune pressure on viral virulence. As previously mentioned, this explains why the threat of a highly virulent lineage causing a huge wave of enhanced severe disease is now imminent in highly vaccinated populations

11.8. Co-circulation of highly infectious Omicron descendants has resulted in diminished viral shedding. Why would these highly infectious variants evolve to become highly virulent rather than highly sheddable/transmissible?

Highly infectious Omicron descendants are forcing the immune system of vaccinated individuals to pair enhanced CTL-mediated inhibition of viral transmissibility with enhanced PNNAb-mediated pressure on viral trans infectiousness/virulence. In a previous contribution (ref. 5) I had described in detail the evolutionary pathway highly infectious Omicron descendants are on the verge of following to select a new variant able to promptly abrogate PNNAb-mediated immune pressure on viral virulence (once this threshold has been breached by highly vaccinated populations). This pathway is the only feasible and rational strategy for the virus to ensure continued viral replication. In contrast, highly infectious variants that would evolve to escape CTL-mediated inhibition of viral transmissibility would be doomed to disappear by killing their host populations.

As the cascade of immune escape events finally resulted in co-circulation of a subset of highly infectious variants, vaccinated individuals with untrained or insufficiently trained CBIIS have now become highly susceptible to Ab-independent VBTIs. These VBTIs allow pre-existing vaccine-induced pNAbs to bind in relatively high concentration to free progeny virus[66] (chapter 3.1.). This is thought to promote clustering of SC-2 virions and thereby stimulate production of Th-independent PNNAbs before the weak viral aggregates are taken up into patrolling APCs to enhance CTL activation (chapter 3.1.). Despite re-stimulation of PNNAbs, the concentration of PNNAbs that bind with low affinity to DC-tethered virions is thought to be diluted at any given time after exposure due to the enhanced adsorption of highly infectious progeny virus onto the surface of these DCs. Under this assumption, it would be reasonable to conclude that upon (re-)exposure to highly infectious Omicron descendants, PNNAbs exert gradually increasing immune pressure on viral *trans* infectiousness while symptoms and shedding/transmission would gradually decline due to enhanced CTL-activity.

In other words, Ab-independent VBTIs would allow more and more SC-2 virions to adsorb to migratory DCs while less and less virus would be shed. To be more specific, at any given time following exposure more and more viruses would be contained within the body of a vaccinated individual.

By introducing a few amino acid mutations in close proximity to the variant-nonspecific antigenic site within S-NTD, the virus could accommodate O-glycosite mutations that enable enhanced *trans* infectiousness of highly infectious progeny virus attached to DCs without making any changes to the conserved antigenic site itself[67] (ref. 5). This is why Nature has shaped this ecosystem in ways that cause the population to exert humoral immune pressure on *viral trans infectiousness* and *not on viral shedding/transmissibility*–the only way for the virus to escape from immune pressure on viral shedding would be to select a mutation that alters the antigenicity of its universal MHC class I-unrestricted CTL peptide. In contrast to S-derived BCR-binding peptides which vary their antigenicity to modulate viral infectiousness, the universal S-derived T cell receptor (TCR)-binding peptide needs to stay highly conserved to universally match all host MHC class I haplotypes (chapter 3.3.). Since this peptide is instrumental in abrogating infection, regardless of the level of intrinsic viral infectiousness, changes to its antigenic constellation would no longer grant a self-limiting nature to coronavirus infections, and for that matter to coronavirus pandemics, without causing large losses of lives in the host population. A high case fatality rate would, however, be counterproductive to viral perpetuation.

11.9. Which immunological mechanism is currently preventing the vast majority of vaccinated individuals from contracting disease upon exposure to more highly infectious co-circulating variants? Does this mechanism interfere with protection against other diseases?

Activation of MHC class I-unrestricted CTLs in vaccinated individuals is now steadily increasing as a result of co-circulation of multiple Omicron descendants that have a high level of intrinsic infectiousness. Enhanced activation of cytolytic capacity towards virus-infected cells strongly mitigates disease symptoms in vaccinated individuals. It is therefore not surprising to find that morbidity rates in vaccinated people have been declining since highly infectious Omicron descendants started to co-circulate[68]. However, as enhanced CTL activity results from enhanced SC-2 virus uptake into professional, tissue-resident APCs, SC-2 increasingly outcompeted other pathogen-derived Ags for uptake and presentation by APCs. Enhanced virus uptake into APCs prevents recall or priming of effector B and T cells that depend on CD4+ T help. This suggests that VBTIs could indirectly downregulate the overall B and T cell repertoire so profoundly that conventional B and T cell responses to peptide pools derived not only from Omicron-derived variants but also from other pathogenic agents are reduced, irrespective of the vaccinated individual's previous infection or vaccination history (refs. 27 and 33). This likely explains the high incidence of other acute infections or re-activation of chronic infectious or noninfectious, immune-mediated diseases and why co-circulating, highly infectious Omicron descendants cannot prime *de novo* immune responses to protect vaccinated individuals via durable, cognate Th-dependent NAbs.

I have not only predicted that immune dysregulation in vaccinated individuals would enhance the pathogenesis of other diseases, but also that it may cause highly vaccinated populations to serve as asymptomatic reservoirs for the transmission of other viral pathogens that generally/commonly cause acute symptomatic infections that are naturally self-limiting (refs. 34-35).

11.10. How do vaccinated individuals manage to largely reduce viral shedding of highly infectious variants even though their immune system cannot recognize these new variants?

As (PNN)Ab-independent VBTIs with highly infectious Omicron descendants no longer enable SIR, and as high intrinsic viral infectiousness compromises APC-mediated stimulation of CD4+ T helper cells, *de novo* immune priming of variant S-specific or cross-functional Abs is no longer possible (chapter 8.2.). As long as vaccinal pNAb titers are sufficiently high, the concentration of these Th-independent PNNAbs is collectively increasing upon re-exposure and thereby reducing viral shedding while slowing the increase in PNNAb-mediated immune pressure on viral virulence.

11.11. Why will vaccine booster doses and expansion of mass vaccination to additional (i.e., younger age groups) only precipitate a public and individual health disaster?

PNNAb-dependent VBTIs bypass the CBIIS and eventually lead to prolonged and widespread immune pressure on viral virulence. Similar to SIR-enabling VBTIs, SIR-enabling mRNA vaccines sideline the CBIIS and promote a cascade of immune escape events that rapidly cause highly vaccinated populations to place high immune pressure on viral virulence.

It is therefore undeniable that high numbers of PNNAb-dependent VBTIs and mRNA-based vaccinations (including mRNA booster doses) together with vaccination of other segments of the population (i.e., including children) have increased the prevalence of SIR events in the population and therefore prevented or abrogated cell-based innate immune training while expediting immune escape. This has led to co-circulation of a diversified set of highly infectious Omicron descendants in highly vaccinated populations.

Even with updated Omicron-adapted vaccines, continued boosting () during exposure to these highly infectious variants will no longer slow the pace at which PNNAb-mediated immune pressure is currently increasing in highly vaccinated populations (chapter 8.2.). One can only conclude that all conditions are now fulfilled for the virus to unleash a global health disaster similar to that which I have been warning about since early 2021.

11.12. Why is the imminent threat of a new emerging, highly virulent variant due to the mass vaccination program?

The cascades of events connecting the mass vaccination program with increasing population-level immune pressure on viral virulence are depicted in the flow diagrams attached (figs. 4 and 8). The event that has undoubtedly triggered this self-catalyzing cascade is rooted in the mass vaccination program. Mass vaccination campaigns that are conducted in the heat of a pandemic cause highly vaccinated populations to place large-scale immune pressure on variant-specific neutralizing epitopes by virtue of a high prevalence of rising titers of high-affinity NAbs that are directed at S variant-specific immunodominant epitopes. Because those Abs need time to fully mature, the immune pressure exerted by the population is suboptimal and will therefore gradually drive immune selection and dominant propagation of more infectious and NAb-evasive lineages.

As the neutralizing capacity of the vaccine-induced pNAbs to S protein expressed on sequentially circulating immune escape variants further diminished, OOV suddenly emerged. This particular and unique immune escape variant had been selected as it had incorporated sufficient S-associated mutations to spectacularly diminish the neutralizing capacity of previously vaccine-primed Abs and provoke PNNAb-mediated VBTIs.

By triggering SIR, PNNAb-mediated VBTIs eventually enabled large-scale immune escape and the emergence of highly infectious variants that are now no longer triggering SIR. Instead, these new emerging variants are triggering Ab-independent VBTIs that result in prolonged suboptimal immune pressure on viral *trans* infectiousness and diminished viral shedding (fig. 6) (chapters 3.1., 3.3. and 6.2.).

Although the immune system of vaccinated individuals can–for now–ensure protection against (severe) disease, this benefit cannot be granted without placing more immune pressure on viral survival. This immune pressure is now rapidly rising in several highly vaccinated countries (as can be concluded from rising hospitalization rates). There can therefore be no doubt that–at this stage of the immune escape pandemic–viral survival will require the blockade on viral virulence to be lifted. The alleged benefits from mass vaccination will likely come at an extraordinary high cost in terms of human lives, predominantly in highly vaccinated countries.

11.13. How (likely) will variants escape from PNNAb-mediated immune pressure on viral virulence?

In a previous contribution, I predicted that SARS-CoV-2 will turn PNNAb-facilitated immune pressure on viral virulence into Ab-independent triggering of enhanced severe/systemic disease. I postulated that this would occur through natural selection of immune escape mutations enabling accommodation of more heavily glycosylated O-glycosite mutations that abolish inhibition of *trans* infection by PNNAbs (ref. 5).

PNNAb-independent VBTIs enable PNNAbs in highly vaccinated populations to establish prolonged and widespread suboptimal immune pressure on viral virulence (i.e., by preventing the conserved enhancing site within S-NTD from facilitating viral *trans* infection). Initially, exposure and re-exposure to currently co-circulating, highly infectious Omicron descendants resulted in a relatively slow increase in PNNAb-mediated immune pressure. This is because the relatively lower binding of PNNAbs to highly concentrated DC-tethered progeny virus was compensated by an enhanced production of PNNAbs as a result of high titers of pre-existing vaccinal pNAbs (chapter 3.1.).

I am convinced that due to a self-extinguishing effect of vaccine booster doses, re-exposure to co-circulating, more infectious variants will eventually lift that blockade before the concomitant reduction of viral shedding in highly vaccinated populations threatens viral survival. It is in my opinion no longer a question of *'if'*, but of *'when'* these variants will emerge.

11.14. Why will society be caught by surprise?

It is important to note that diminished protection against productive infection normally implies lowered protection against viral virulence. With the advent of Omicron, however, this relationship has been inverted– enhanced viral infectiousness resulted in protection against (i.e., severe) disease. This is because PNNAbs not only enhanced viral infectiousness (i.e., due to the diminished neutralizability of Omicron), but also presumably prevented *trans* infection (and hence, *trans* fusion) of progeny virions adsorbed onto migratory DCs (ref. 5). Large-scale circulation of highly infectious Omicron descendants is now fostering PNNAb-independent VBTIs in vaccinated individuals. As explained in chapters 3.1., 3.3. and 3.9, this promotes uptake of pNAb-complexed virions into tissue-resident DCs/APCs and thereby enhances cytolytic clearance of virus-infected host cells (fig. 11). This not only results in diminished viral shedding but also mitigation of disease symptoms. In vaccinated individuals, the durability of this inverted relationship will only hold until enhanced adsorption of highly infectious progeny virus increases PNNAb-mediated immune pressure above a threshold necessary to drive natural selection of an immune escape variant capable of lifting the blockade imposed by PNNAbs on viral virulence in the majority of the vaccinated population.

While *de facto* reflecting the 'calm before the tsunami', this inverted relationship is currently obfuscating the imminent threat the ongoing evolutionary dynamics are posing to vaccinated individuals in highly vaccinated countries.

11.15. How will the immune escape pandemic end for vaccinated individuals, unvaccinated individuals, and.... for the virus? (figs. 4, 8 and 9)

Whereas herd immunity curtails transmission and rapidly abrogates morbidity and mortality rates, herd immune pressure on infectiousness and virulence can only curtail transmission by provoking a spectacular rise in mortality rates in vaccinated populations. In highly vaccinated countries this rise is preceded by an increased hospitalization rate in vaccinated individuals that is due to other acute and chronic infectious, inflammatory or immune-mediated diseases

(Re-)exposure to steadily co-emerging and co-circulating Omicron descendants exhibiting high intrinsic infectiousness is now forcing vaccinated individuals to breed new variants that are likely to lead to enhanced severe disease. In contrast, similar exposure of healthy unvaccinated individuals to these highly infectious variants will serve to further assist CBIIS training (mostly following some mild symptoms). This is critically important to maintain robust protection against Ab-independent BTIs caused by highly infectious Omicron descendants, some of which are already more virulent. As new emerging Omicron-derived variants will no longer be selected for enhanced infectiousness, but enhanced virulence, unvaccinated individuals with adequate CBIIS training should even be protected from disease altogether. So long as the virus is evolving to acquire more virulent properties, it will be important for the unvaccinated and vaccinated individuals whose CBIIS training has not yet been compromised by vaccination to maintain some level of exposure[69] in order to preserve strong cell-based sterilizing immune capacity.

At this stage of the pandemic, virus adaptation to the immune status of a highly vaccinated population requires immune escape variants to evade the virulence-inhibiting activity of PNNAbs. Gradually increasing population-level immune pressure on viral virulence will eventually surge to enable selection of a highly virulent immune escape variant that is likely to separately provoke an impressive wave of hospitalization and death in highly vaccinated countries. Until now, enhanced hospitalization rates in vaccinated individuals were primarily due to an increased incidence of other acute and chronic infectious, inflammatory or immune-mediated diseases[70].

I postulate that the combination of a high hospitalization and mortality rate in the vaccinated cohort of a highly vaccinated population, together with the high sterilizing capacity rendered by the CBIIS of the unvaccinated will rapidly entail eradication of such new emerging, highly virulent virus (herein called 'HIVICRON'). It is uncertain whether prophylactic treatment with antivirals would prevent vaccinated individuals from contracting AIESD or possibly curtail productive infection and shedding of variants with such enhanced intrinsic infectiousness and virulence.

Whereas high case fatality rates will need to bring the pandemic to an end in highly vaccinated countries, countries/regions with a low vaccine coverage rates could primarily rely on herd immunity to end the pandemic, provided they stop the vaccination program. This would allow these countries to rapidly and drastically reduce population-level immune pressure on viral virulence while allowing the unvaccinated part of the population to diminish viral transmission via herd immunity. However, it is clear that even in countries with relatively low vaccination rates, the toll on human lives could still be relatively high. This is because abrogation of the vaccination program will leave vaccinated individuals without PNNAbs to protect them from severe disease. Given the deficient/insufficient training of their CBIIS and the enhanced intrinsic infectiousness of co-circulating variants (mostly not more virulent), many vaccinated individuals may contract severe disease (but not 'enhanced' severe disease).

Of course, in countries/regions with lower vaccine coverage rates the combination of enhanced mortality rate with substantial herd immunity could potentially be complemented by antivirals to reduce viral transmission more rapidly. Early multidrug treatment could save lives of vaccinated individuals while helping patients to contribute to herd immunity. Given the high level of efficiency of herd immunity and mortality in reducing viral transmission, it is likely that the virus will ultimately be eradicated. However, it is not until eradication occurs in all vaccinated countries that this immune escape pandemic can be terminated globally.

11.16. Why should no single individual have been motivated, let alone coerced, to take the vaccine?

Vaccinated individuals breed immune escape variants that are more and more infectious. While this initially rendered the unvaccinated more susceptible to contracting disease (including disease resulting from PNNAb-dependent NBTI with Omicron), adapted cell-mediated immune training following re-infection is now lowering the likelihood for an unvaccinated person to develop disease (including disease caused by PNNAb-dependent BTI). However, infection with Omicron in vaccine-primed individuals has prevented or even abrogated immune training of innate immune cells. This is because exposure to Omicron in the presence of pre-existing vaccine-induced pNAbs with low neutralizing capacity triggered SIR-enabling VBTIs. In addition, SIR-enabling VBTIs with early Omicron descendants have been paving the way to the emergence and co-circulation of highly infectious Omicron descendants which cause widespread Ab-independent VBTIs in highly vaccinated populations. The latter are now enabling gradually increasing PNNAb-mediated immune pressure on viral virulence in vaccinated individuals. This is now generating a life-threatening situation for many vaccinated individuals in highly vaccinated countries/regions.

No single individual should therefore have received vaccines. Healthy unvaccinated individuals who regularly experienced productive infection–and therefore have a trained CBIIS endowed with strong sterilizing immune capacity–will ultimately perform much better than their vaccinated peers. Not only will their trained CBIIS greatly improve their individual immune protection against disease, but they also critically contribute to preventing viral transmission and establishing herd immunity without driving immune escape. It has therefore been a major blunder to convince anyone of vaccination during a pandemic. Even individuals with a frail CBIIS (e.g., elderly, those with comorbidities or otherwise immune suppressed) should not have received vaccines but rather allowed prophylactic antiviral or early multidrug treatment.

References

These references support the insights and hypothesis presented in this book. Please also find a nonexhaustive list of references associated with this book online at https://www.voiceforscienceandsolidarity.org/blog/resources-accompanying-my-book or by scanning this QR Code.

Literature References

1. Kulkarni R. (2019). *Antibody-Dependent Enhancement of Viral Infections*. Dynamics of Immune Activation in Viral Diseases, 9–41.
https://doi.org/10.1007/978-981-15-1045-8_2\
https://www.ncbi.nlm.nih.gov/pmc/articles/PMC711996 4/

2. Liu Y, Soh WT, Kishikawa JI, Hirose M, Nakayama EE, Li S, Sasai M, Suzuki T, Tada A, Arakawa A, Matsuoka S, Akamatsu K, Matsuda M, Ono C, Torii S, Kishida K, Jin H, Nakai W, Arase N, Nakagawa A, Matsumoto M, Nakazaki Y, Shindo Y, Kohyama M, Tomii K, Ohmura K, Ohshima S, Okamoto T, Yamamoto M, Nakagami H, Matsuura Y, Nakagawa A, Kato T, Okada M, Standley DM, Shioda T, Arase H. *An infectivity-enhancing site on the SARS-CoV-2 spike protein targeted by antibodie*s. Cell. 2021 Jun 24;184(13):3452-3466.e18. doi: 10.1016/j.cell.2021.05.032. Epub 2021 May 24. PMID: 34139176; PMCID: PMC8142859.
https://www.ncbi.nlm.nih.gov/pmc/articles/PMC814285 9/

3. Li, D., Edwards, R. J., Manne, K., Martinez, D. R., Schäfer, A., Alam, S. M., Wiehe, K., Lu, X., Parks, R., Sutherland, L. L., Oguin, T. H., 3rd, McDanal, C., Perez, L. G., Mansouri, K., Gobeil, S. M. C., Janowska, K., Stalls, V., Kopp, M., Cai, F., Lee, E., … Saunders, K. O. (2021). *In vitro and in vivo functions of SARS-CoV-2 infection-enhancing and neutralizing antibodies*. Cell, 184(16), 4203–4219.e32.
https://doi.org/10.1016/j.cell.2021.06.021
https://www.ncbi.nlm.nih.gov/pmc/articles/PMC823296 9/

4. Yahi, N., Chahinian, H., & Fantini, J. (2021). *Infection-enhancing anti-SARS-CoV-2 antibodies recognize both the original Wuhan/D614G strain and Delta variants. A*

potential risk for mass vaccination?. The Journal of
infection, *83*(5), 607–635.
  https://doi.org/10.1016/j.jinf.2021.08.010
  https://pubmed.ncbi.nlm.nih.gov/34384810/

5. Vanden Bossche, G. (2022). **Predictions on evolution Covid
19 pandemic**.
  https://www.voiceforscienceandsolidarity.org/scientific-
  blog/predictions-gvb-on-evolution-c-19-pandemic

6. Wu, L., Zhou, L., Mo, M. et al. **SARS-CoV-2 Omicron RBD
shows weaker binding affinity than the currently
dominant Delta variant to human ACE2**. Sig Transduct
Target Ther 7, 8 (2022). https://doi.org/10.1038/s41392-
021-00863-2
  https://www.nature.com/articles/s41392-021-00863-2

7. Tian, W., Li, D., Zhang, N. et al. **O-glycosylation pattern of
the SARS-CoV-2 spike protein reveals an "O-Follow-N"
rule**. Cell Res 31, 1123–1125 (2021).
  https://doi.org/10.1038/s41422-021-00545-2
  https://www.nature.com/articles/s41422-021-00545-2

8. Watanabe, Y., Bowden, T. A., Wilson, I. A., & Crispin, M.
(2019). **Exploitation of glycosylation in enveloped virus
pathobiology**. Biochimica et biophysica acta. General
subjects, *1863*(10), 1480–1497.
  https://doi.org/10.1016/j.bbagen.2019.05.012
  https://www.ncbi.nlm.nih.gov/pmc/articles/PMC668607
  7/

9. Shajahan, A., Supekar, N.T., Gleinich, A.S., Azadi, P., (2020)
**Deducing the N- and O-glycosylation profile of the spike
protein of novel coronavirus SARS-CoV-2**. Glycobiology, ,
Volume 30, Issue 12, December 2020, Pages 981–988.
  https://www.ncbi.nlm.nih.gov/pmc/articles/PMC723918
  3/pdf/cwaa042.pdf)

10. Kull, K., (2000), *Organisms can be proud to have been their own designers*. Cybernetics & Human Knowing, Volume 7, Number 1, 1 January 2000, pp. 45-55(11). https://www.ingentaconnect.com/content/imp/chk/2000/00000007/00000001/54

11. Taubenberger, J. K., & Morens, D. M. (2006). *1918 Influenza: the mother of all pandemics*. Emerging *infectious diseases*, *12*(1), 15–22. https://doi.org/10.3201/eid1201.050979 https://www.ncbi.nlm.nih.gov/pmc/articles/PMC3291398/pdf/05-0979.pdf

12. Patrono, L.V., Vrancken, B., Budt, M. *et al. Archival influenza virus genomes from Europe reveal genomic variability during the 1918 pandemic*. Nat Commun 13, 2314 (2022). https://doi.org/10.1038/s41467-022-29614-9 https://www.nature.com/articles/s41467-022-29614-9

Within these 57 literature references, 13-32 are a special list (non-exhaustive) of supportive evidence that I used to develop and validate his hypothesis in this book.

13. Quandt, J., Muik, A., Salisch, N., Lui, B. G., Lutz, S., Krüger, K., Wallisch, A. K., Adams-Quack, P., Bacher, M., Finlayson, A., Ozhelvaci, O., Vogler, I., Grikscheit, K., Hoehl, S., Goetsch, U., Ciesek, S., Türeci, Ö., & Sahin, U. (2022). *Omicron BA.1 breakthrough infection drives cross-variant neutralization and memory B cell formation against conserved epitopes*. Science immunology, 7(75), eabq2427. https://doi.org/10.1126/sciimmunol.abq2427 https://pubmed.ncbi.nlm.nih.gov/35653438/

14. Wang, Q., Guo, Y., Iketani, S. *et al*. ***Antibody evasion by SARS-CoV-2 Omicron subvariants BA.2.12.1, BA.4 and BA.5***. *Nature* 608, 603–608 (2022).
https://doi.org/10.1038/s41586-022-05053-w
https://www.nature.com/articles/s41586-022-05053-w

15. Kaku, C. I., Bergeron, A. J., Ahlm, C., Normark, J., Sakharkar, M., Forsell, M. N. E., & Walker, L. M. (2022). ***Recall of preexisting cross-reactive B cell memory after Omicron BA.1 breakthrough infection***. *Science immunology*, *7*(73), eabq3511.
https://doi.org/10.1126/sciimmunol.abq3511
https://www.ncbi.nlm.nih.gov/pmc/articles/PMC909788 2/

16. Nutalai, R., Zhou, D., Tuekprakhon, A., Ginn, H. M., Supasa, P., Liu, C., Huo, J., Mentzer, A. J., Duyvesteyn, H. M. E., Dijokaite-Guraliuc, A., Skelly, D., Ritter, T. G., Amini, A., Bibi, S., Adele, S., Johnson, S. A., Constantinides, B., Webster, H., Temperton, N., Klenerman, P., ... Screaton, G. R. (2022). ***Potent cross-reactive antibodies following Omicron breakthrough in vaccinees***. *Cell*, *185*(12), 2116–2131.e18.
https://doi.org/10.1016/j.cell.2022.05.014
https://www.ncbi.nlm.nih.gov/pmc/articles/PMC912013 0/

17. Arora, P., Kempf, A., Nehlmeier, I., Schulz, S.R., Cossmann, A., Metodi V Stankov, M.V., Hans-Martin Jäck, H.M., Georg M N Behrens, G.M.N., Stefan Pöhlmann, S., Markus Hoffmann, M., (2022), ***Augmented neutralisation resistance of emerging omicron subvariants BA.2.12.1, BA.4, and BA.5***., The Lancet, Volume 22, Issue 8, August 2022, Pages 1117-1118, https://doi.org/10.1016/S1473-3099(22)00422-4.
https://www.thelancet.com/action/showPdf?pii=S1473-3099%2822%2900422-4

18. Wratil, P.R., Stern, M., Priller, A. *et al.*, (2022), ***Three exposures to the spike protein of SARS-CoV-2 by either infection or vaccination elicit superior neutralizing immunity to all variants of concern***. Nat Med 28, 496–503.
https://doi.org/10.1038/s41591-022-01715-4
https://www.nature.com/articles/s41591-022-01715-4

19. Muecksch, F., Wang, Z., Cho, A. *et al.*, (2022), ***Increased memory B cell potency and breadth after a SARS-CoV-2 mRNA boost***. *Nature* 607, 128–134.
https://doi.org/10.1038/s41586-022-04778-y
https://www.nature.com/articles/s41586-022-04778-y

20. Munro, A. P. S., Janani, L., Cornelius, V., Aley, P. K., Babbage, G., Baxter, D., Bula, M., Cathie, K., Chatterjee, K., Dodd, K., Enever, Y., Gokani, K., Goodman, A. L., Green, C. A., Harndahl, L., Haughney, J., Hicks, A., van der Klaauw, A. A., Kwok, J., Lambe, T., COV-BOOST study group (2021). ***Safety and immunogenicity of seven COVID-19 vaccines as a third dose (booster) following two doses of ChAdOx1 nCov-19 or BNT162b2 in the UK (COV-BOOST): a blinded, multicentre, randomized, controlled, phase 2 trial***. *Lancet (London, England)*, *398*(10318), 2258–2276.
https://doi.org/10.1016/S0140-6736(21)02717-3
https://www.ncbi.nlm.nih.gov/pmc/articles/PMC8639161/

21. Fanchong Jian, Yuanling Yu, Weiliang Song, Ayijiang Yisimayi, Lingling Yu, Yuxue Gao, Na Zhang, Yao WangFei Shao, Xiaohua Hao, Yanli Xu, Ronghua Jin, Youchun Wang, Xiaoliang Sunney Xie, Yunlong Cao, (2022), ***Further humoral immunity evasion of emerging SARS-CoV-2 BA.4 and BA.5 subvariants***, volume 22, issue 11, P1535-1537.
https://doi.org/10.1016/S1473-3099(22)00642-9

https://www.biorxiv.org/content/10.1101/2022.08.09.50
3384v1.full.pdf

22. Sugano, A., Takaoka, Y., Kataguchi, H., Kumaoka, M., Ohta,
M., Kimura, S., Araki, M., Morinaga, Y., Yamamoto, Y.,
(2022), *SARS-CoV-2 Omicron BA.2.75 variant may be
much more infective than preexisting variant*
https://doi.org/10.1101/2022.08.25.505217
https://www.biorxiv.org/content/10.1101/2022.08.25.50
5217v4.full.pdf

23. Cao, Y., Jian, F., Wang, J., Yu, Y. Song, W., Yisimayi, A., Wang,
J., An, R. Chen, X., Zhang, N., Wang, Y. Wang, P. Zhao, L., Sun,
H., Yu, L., Yang, S., Niu, X., Xiao, T., Gu, Q., Shao, F., Hao, X.,
Xu, Y., Jin, R., Shen, Z., Wang, Y., Xie, X.S., (2022), *Imprinted
SARS-CoV-2 humoral immunity induces convergent
Omicron RBD evolution*.
https://doi.org/10.1101/2022.09.15.507787
https://www.biorxiv.org/content/10.1101/2022.09.15.50
7787v4.full.pdf

24. Starr, T.N., Greaney, A.J., Stewart, C.M., Walls, A.C., Hannon,
W.W., Veesler, D., Bloom, J.D., (2022), *Deep mutational
scans for ACE2 binding, RBD expression, and antibody
escape in the SARS-CoV-2 Omicron BA.1 and BA.2
receptor-binding domains*., PLoS Pathog 18(11):
e1010951.
https://doi.org/10.1371/journal.ppat.1010951.
https://www.biorxiv.org/content/10.1101/2022.09.20.50
8745v1.full.pdf

25. Muik, A., Lui, B.G., Bacher,, M., Wallisch, A-K., Toker, A.,
Finlayson, A., Krüger, K., Ozhelvaci, O., Grikscheit, K., Hoehl,
S., Ciesek, S., Türeci, Ö., Sahin, U., (2022), *Omicron BA.2
breakthrough infection enhances cross-neutralization
of BA.2.12.1 and BA.4/BA.5*., Science Immunology, Vol 7,
Issue 77, DOI: 10.1126/sciimmunol.ade2283.

https://www.science.org/doi/epdf/10.1126/sciimmunol.ade2283

26. Cao, Y., Yisimayi, A., Jian, F. *et al.,* (2022), ***BA.2.12.1, BA.4 and BA.5 escape antibodies elicited by Omicron infection***. Nature 608, 593–602. https://doi.org/10.1038/s41586-022-04980-y https://www.nature.com/articles/s41586-022-04980-y

27. Reynolds, C. J., Pade, C., Gibbons, J. M., Otter, A. D., Lin, K. M., Muñoz Sandoval, D., Pieper, F. P., Butler, D. K., Liu, S., Joy, G., Forooghi, N., Treibel, T. A., Manisty, C., Moon, J. C., COVIDsortium Investigators§, COVIDsortium Immune Correlates Network§, Semper, A., Brooks, T., McKnight, Á., Altmann, D. M., Moon, J. C. (2022). ***Immune boosting by B.1.1.529 (Omicron) depends on previous SARS-CoV-2 exposure***. Science *(New York, N.Y.)*, *377*(6603), eabq1841. https://doi.org/10.1126/science.abq1841. https://www.ncbi.nlm.nih.gov/pmc/articles/PMC9210451/

28. Hoffmann, M., Krüger, N., Schulz, S., Cossmann, A., Rocha, C., Kempf, A., Nehlmeier, I., Graichen, L., Moldenhauer, A.-S., Winkler, M.S., Lier, M., Dopfer-Jablonka, A., Jäck, H-m., Behrens, G.M.N., (2022), ***The Omicron variant is highly resistant against antibody-mediated neutralization: Implications for control of the COVID-19 pandemic***, Cell, Volume 185, Issue 3, Pages 447-456.e11, https://doi.org/10.1016/j.cell.2021.12.032 https://www.sciencedirect.com/science/article/pii/S0092867421014951

29. Irrgang, P. Gerling, J., Kocher, K., Lapuente, D., Steininger, P., Habenicht, K., Wytopil, ., Beileke, S., Schäfer, S., Zhong, J., Ssebyatika, G., Krey, T., Falcone, V., Schïmein, C., Peter, A.S. Nganou-Makamdop, K., Hengel, H., Held, J., Bogdan, C. Überla, K., Schober, K., Winkler, T.H., Tenbusch, M., (2022),

Class switch towards non-inflammatory, spike-specific IgG4 antibodies after repeated SARS-CoV-2 mRNA vaccination, DOI: 10.1126/sciimmunol.ade279.https://www.science.org/doi/10.1126/sciimmunol.ade2798

30. Witte, L., Baharani, V., Schmidt, F., Wang, Z., Cho, A., Raspe, R., Guzman-Cardozo, M.C., Muecksch, F., Gaebler, C., Caskey, M., Nussenzweig, M.C., Hatziioannou, T., Bieniasz, P.D., (2022), *Epistasis lowers the genetic barrier to SARS-CoV-2 neutralizing antibody escape.* https://doi.org/10.1101/2022.08.17.504313 https://www.biorxiv.org/content/10.1101/2022.08.17.504313v1.full.pdf

31. Kaku, C.I., Starr, T.N., Zhou, P., Dugan, H.L., Khalifé, P., Song, G., Champney, E.R., Mielcarz, D.W., Geoghegan, J.C., Burton, D.R., Andrabi, R., Bloom, J.D., Walker, L.M., (2022), *Evolution of antibody immunity following Omicron BA.1 breakthrough infection.* https://doi.org/10.1101/2022.09.21.508922 https://www.biorxiv.org/content/10.1101/2022.09.21.508922v1.full.pdf

32. Muik, A., Lui, B.G., Bacher, M., Wallisch, A.-K., Toker, A. Finlayson, A. Krüger, K., Ozhelvaci, O., Grikscheit, K., Hoehl, S., Ciesek, S., Türeci, Ö., Sahin, U., (2022), *Omicron BA.2 breakthrough infection enhances cross-neutralization of BA.2.12.1 and BA.4/BA.5.*, https://doi.org/10.1101/2022.08.02.502461 https://www.biorxiv.org/content/10.1101/2022.08.02.502461v1.full.pdf

33. Vanden Bossche, G., (2022), *Immuno-epidemiologic ramifications of the C-19 mass vaccination experiment: Individual and global health consequences.* www.voiceforscienceandsolidarity.org/scientific-

blog/immuno-epidemiologic-ramifications-of-the-c-19-mass-vaccination-experiment-individual-and-global-health-consequences

34. Vanden Bossche, G., (2022), *Instead of generating herd immunity, C-19 mass vaccination triggers a chain reaction of new pandemics and epidemics.* https://www.voiceforscienceandsolidarity.org/scientific-blog/c-19-mass-vaccination-triggers-a-chain-reaction-of-new-pandemics-and-epidemics.

35. Vanden Bossche, G., (2022), *A Fairy Tale of Pandemics*. https://www.voiceforscienceandsolidarity.org/scientific-blog/a-fairy-tale-of-pandemics

36. Collier, A.Y., Miller, J., Hachmann, N.P., McMahan, K., Liu, J., Apraku Bondzie, E., Gallup, L., Rowe, M., Schonberg, E., Thai, S., Barrett, J., Borducchi, E.N., Bouffard, E., Jacob-Dolan, C., Mazurek, C.R., Mutoni, A., Powers, O., Sciacca, M., Surve, N., VanWyk, H., Wu, C., Barouch, D.H., (2022), *Immunogenicity of the BA.5 Bivalent mRNA Vaccine Boosters*. https://doi.org/10.1101/2022.10.24.513619 https://www.biorxiv.org/content/10.1101/2022.10.24.513619v1.full.pdf

37. Wang, Q., Bowen, A., Valdez, R., Gherasim, C., Gordon, A., Liu L., Ho, D.D., (2022), *Antibody responses to Omicron BA.4/BA.5 bivalent mRNA vaccine booster shot.*, https://doi.org/10.1101/2022.10.22.513349 https://www.biorxiv.org/content/10.1101/2022.10.22.513349v1.full.pdf

38. Collier, A.Y., Miller, J., Hachmann, N.P., McMahan, K., Liu, J., Bondzie, E.A., Gallup, L., Rowe, M., Schonberg, E., Thai, S., Barrett, J., Borducchi, E.N., Bouffard, E., Jacob-Dolan, C., Mazurek, C.R. Mutoni, A., Powers, O., Sciacca, M., Surve, N.,

VanWyk, H., Wu, C., Barouch, D.H., (2023),
***Immunogenicity of BA.5 Bivalent mRNA Vaccine
Boosters***, New England Journal of Medicine,
10.1056/NEJMc2213948.
https://www.nejm.org/doi/pdf/10.1056/NEJMc2213948?
articleTools=true

39. Vanden Bossche, G., (2022), Novel bivalent C-19 vaccines:
***What does common immunological sense predict in
regard to their impact on the C-19 pandemic?***
https://www.voiceforscienceandsolidarity.org/scientific-
blog/novel-bivalent-c-19-vaccines-what-does-common-
immunological-sense-predict-in-regard-to-their-impact-
on-the-c-19-pandemic.

40. Lempp, F.A., Soriaga, L.B., Montiel-Ruiz, M., Benigni, F.,
Noack, J., Park, Y-J., Bianchi, S., Walls, A.C., Bowen, J.E. Zhou,
J., Kaiser, H., Joshi, A., Agostini, M., Meury, M., Dellota, E Jr.,
Jaconi, S., Cameroni, E., Martinez-Picado, J., Vergara-Alert,
J., Izquierdo-Useros, N., Virgin, H. W., Lanzavecchia, A.,
Veesler, D., Purcell, L. A. Telenti, A., Corti, D., (2021),
***Lectins enhance SARS-CoV-2 infection and influence
neutralizing antibodies.***
https://doi.org/10.1038/s41586-021-03925-1
https://www.nature.com/articles/s41586-021-03925-
1.pdf

41-42. Perez-Zsolt, D., Muñoz-Basagoiti, J., Rodon, J., Elosua-
Bayes, M., Raïch-Regué, D., Risco, C., Sachse, M., Pino, M.,
Gumber, S., Paiardini, M., Chojnacki, J., Erkizia, I., Muñiz-
Trabudua, X., Ballana, E., Riveira-Muñoz, E., Noguera-
Julian, M., Paredes, R., Trinité, B., Tarrés-Freixas, F., Blanco,
I., ... Izquierdo-Useros, N. (2021). ***SARS-CoV-2 interaction
with Siglec-1 mediates trans-infection by dendritic cells***.
Cellular & molecular immunology, 18(12), 2676–2678.
https://doi.org/10.1038/s41423-021-00794-6
https://pubmed.ncbi.nlm.nih.gov/34782760/

https://doi.org/10.1101/2021.05.11.443572

43. Vanden Bossche, G., (2021), *When anti-S(pike) antibodies against Omicron can no longer sustain the narrative, why not resort to T cells?* https://www.voiceforscienceandsolidarity.org/scientific-blog/when-anti-s-pike-antibodies-against-omicron-can-no-longer-sustain-the-narrative-why-not-resort-to-t-cells

44. Madu, I. G., Roth, S. L., Belouzard, S., & Whittaker, G. R. (2009). *Characterization of a highly conserved domain within the severe acute respiratory syndrome coronavirus spike protein S2 domain with characteristics of a viral fusion peptide.* Journal of virology, 83(15), 7411–7421. https://doi.org/10.1128/JVI.00079-09.

https://www.ncbi.nlm.nih.gov/pmc/articles/PMC2708636/

45. Lin, D. Y., Gu, Y., Xu, Y., Zeng, D., Wheeler, B., Young, H., Sunny, S. K., & Moore, Z. (2022). *Effects of Vaccination and Previous Infection on Omicron Infections in Children.* The New England journal of medicine, 387(12), 1141–1143. https://doi.org/10.1056/NEJMc2209371 https://pubmed.ncbi.nlm.nih.gov/36069811/

46. Agerer, B., Koblischke, M., Gudipati, V., Montaño-Gutierrez, L. F., Smyth, M., Popa, A., Genger, J. W., Endler, L., Florian, D. M., Mühlgrabner, V., Graninger, M., Aberle, S. W., Husa, A. M., Shaw, L. E., Lercher, A., Gattinger, P., Torralba-Gombau, R., Trapin, D., Penz, T., Barreca, D., ... Bergthaler, A. (2021). *SARS-CoV-2 mutations in MHC-I-restricted epitopes evade CD8+ T cell responses.* Science immunology, 6(57), eabg6461.

https://doi.org/10.1126/sciimmunol.abg6461
https://pubmed.ncbi.nlm.nih.gov/33664060/

47. Dolton, G., Rius, C., Hasan, S., Wall, A., Szomolay, B., Behiry, E., Whalley, T., Southgate, J., Fuller, A., Morin, T., Topley, K., Rong Tan, L., Goulder, P.J.R., Spiller, O.B., Rizkallah, P.J., Jones, L.C., Connor, T.R., Sewell, A.K., (2022), *Emergence of immune escape at dominant SARS-CoV-2 killer T cell epitope.*, Cell, Volume 185, Issue 16, Pages 2936-2951.e19. https://doi.org/10.1016/j.cell.2022.07.002. https://www.sciencedirect.com/science/article/p ii/S0092867422008492

48. Kimura, I., Yamasoba, D., Tamura, T., Nao, N., Suzuki, T., Oda, Y., Mitoma, S., Ito, J., Nasser, H., Zahradnik, J., Uriu, K., Fujita, S., Kosugi, Y., Wang, L., Tsuda, M., Kishimoto, M., Ito, H., Suzuki, R., Shimizu, R., Begum, M. M., ... Sato, K. (2022). *Virological characteristics of the SARS-CoV-2 Omicron BA.2 subvariants, including BA.4 and BA.5.* Cell, *185*(21), 3992–4007.e16. https://doi.org/10.1016/j.cell.2022.09.018.

https://www.biorxiv.org/content/10.1101/2022.12.27.52 1986v1.full.pdf

49. Saito, A., Irie, T., Suzuki, R., Maemura, T., Nasser, H., Uriu, K., Kosugi, Y., Shirakawa, K., Sadamasu, K., Kimura, I., Ito, J., Wu, J., Iwatsuki-Horimoto, K., Ito, M., Yamayoshi, S., Ozono, S., Erika PButlertanaka, Tanaka, Y.L., Shimizu, R., Shimizu, K., Yoshimatsu, K., RyokoKawabata, Sakaguchi, T., Tokunaga, K., Yoshida, I., Asakura, H., Nagashima, M., Kazuma, Y., Nomura, R., Horisawa, Y., Yoshimura, K., Takaori-Kondo, A., Imai, M., The Genotype to Phenotype Japan (G2P-Japan) Consortium, Nakagawa, S. Ikeda, T., Fukuhara, T., Kawaoka, Y., Sato, K., (2021), *SARS-CoV-2 spike P681R mutation, a hallmark of the Delta variant, enhances viral fusogenicity and pathogenicity.*, ioRxiv

2021.06.17.448820; doi:
https://doi.org/10.1101/2021.06.17.448820
https://www.biorxiv.org/content/10.1101/2021.06.17.44
8820v1.full.pdf

50. Qu, P., Faraone, J.N., Evans, J.P., Zou, X., Zheng, Y., Carlin, C.,
Bednash, J.S., Lozanski, G., Mallampalli, R.K., Saif, L.J., Oltz,
E.M., Mohler, P.J., Gumina, R.J., Liu, S., (2022), *Differential
Evasion of Delta and Omicron Immunity and Enhanced
Fusogenicity of SARS-CoV-2 Omicron BA.4/5 and
BA.2.12.1 Subvariants., bioRxiv 2022.05.16.492158; doi:
https://doi.org/10.1101/2022.05.16.492158*
https://www.biorxiv.org/content/10.1101/2022.05.16.49
2158v1.full.pdf

51. Kimura, I., Yamasoba, D., Tamura, T., Nao, N., Suzuki, T.,
Oda, Y., Mitoma, S., Ito, J., Nasser, H., Zahradnik, J., Uriu, K.,
Fujita, S., Kosugi, Y., Wang, L., Tsuda, M., Kishimoto, M., Ito,
H., Suzuki, R., Shimizu, R., Begum, M. M., … Sato, K. (2022).
*Virological characteristics of the SARS-CoV-2 Omicron
BA.2 subvariants, including BA.4 and BA.5*. Cell, *185*(21),
3992–4007.e16.
https://doi.org/10.1016/j.cell.2022.09.018
https://www.cell.com/action/showPdf?pii=S0092-
8674%2822%2901190-4

52. Chumakov, K., Avidan, M. S., Benn, C. S., Bertozzi, S. M., Blatt,
L., Chang, A. Y., Jamison, D. T., Khader, S. A., Kottilil, S.,
Netea, M. G., Sparrow, A., & Gallo, R. C. (2021). *Old
vaccines for new infections: Exploiting innate immunity
to control COVID-19 and prevent future pandemics*.
Proceedings of the National Academy of Sciences of the
United States of America, *118*(21), e2101718118.
https://doi.org/10.1073/pnas.2101718118
https://www.ncbi.nlm.nih.gov/pmc/articles/PMC816616
6/

53. Parmar, K., Siddiqui, A., & Nugent, K. (2021). *Bacillus Calmette-Guerin Vaccine and Non Specific Immunity*. *The American journal of the medical sciences*, *361*(6), 683–689.
https://doi.org/10.1016/j.amjms.2021.03.003
https://www.ncbi.nlm.nih.gov/pmc/articles/PMC793818 9/

54. Brogna, C., Brogna, B., Bisaccia, D. R., Lauritano, F., Marino, G., Montano, L., Cristoni, S., Prisco, M., & Piscopo, M. (2022). *Could SARS-CoV-2 Have Bacteriophage Behavior or Induce the Activity of Other Bacteriophages?*. *Vaccines*, *10*(5), 708.
https://doi.org/10.3390/vaccines10050708
https://www.ncbi.nlm.nih.gov/pmc/articles/PMC914343 5/

55. Li, L., Han, P., Huang, B.et al., (2022), *Broader-species receptor binding and structural bases of Omicron SARS-CoV-2 to both mouse and palm-civet ACE2s*. Cell Discov **8**, 65,
https://doi.org/10.1038/s41421-022-00431-0
https://www.nature.com/articles/s41421-022-00431-0

56. Qu, P., Faraone, J.N., Evans, J.P., Zou, X., Zheng, Y.-M., Carlin, C., Bednash, J.S., Lozanski, G., Mallampalli, R.K., Saif, L.J., Oltz, E.M., Mohler, P.J., Gumina, R.J., Liu, S.-L., (2022), *Differential Evasion of Delta and Omicron Immunity and Enhanced Fusogenicity of SARS-CoV-2 Omicron BA.4/5 and BA.2.12.1 Subvariants*,
https://doi.org/10.1101/2022.05.16.492158
https://www.biorxiv.org/content/10.1101/2022.05.16.49 2158v1.full.pdf

57. Arora, P., Cossmann, A., Schulz, S.R., Morillas Ramos, G., Stankov, M.V., Jäck, H-M., Behrens, G.M.N., Pöhlmann, S., Hoffmann, M., (2023), *Neutralisation sensitivity of the SARS-CoV-2 XBB.1 lineage.*, The Lancet, DOI:

https://doi.org/10.1016/S1473-3099(22)00831-3

https://www.thelancet.com/action/showPdf?pii=S1473-3099%2822%2900831-3

Further Reading

Please visit the designated page of our website at https://www.voiceforscienceandsolidarity.org/blog/resources-accompanying-my-book for additional reading on topics specifically related to this book or scan the QR Code below.

"The greatest enemy in the control of the pandemic is the immunological ignorance of our leading scientific, public health and regulatory experts."

Read here:
https://www.voiceforscienceandsolidarity.org/scientific-blog/the-greatest-enemy-in-the-control-of-the-pandemic-is-the-immunological-ignorance-of-our-leading-scientific-public-health-and-regulatory-experts

"C-19 Pandemia: Quo vadis, homo sapiens?"

Read here:
www.voiceforscienceandsolidarity.org/scientific-blog/c-19-pandemia-quo-vadis-homo-sapiens

"Continued mass vaccination will only push the evolutionary capacity of SARS-CoV-2 Spike protein beyond the Omicron version."

Read here:
www.voiceforscienceandsolidarity.org/scientific-blog/mass-vaccination-will-push-sars-cov-2-spike-protein-beyond-omicron

"A last word of caution to all those pretending the Covid-19 pandemic is toning down..."

Read here:
https://www.voiceforscienceandsolidarity.org/scientific-blog/a-last-word-of-caution-to-all-those-pretending-the-covid-19-pandemic-is-toning-down

"Omicron is not what was initially considered a mysterious blessing…"

Read here:
www.voiceforscienceandsolidarity.org/scientific-blog/omicron-is-not-what-was-initially-considered-a-mysterious-blessing

"Will mass vaccination against Omicron give the final blow?"

Read here:
www.voiceforscienceandsolidarity.org/scientific-blog/will-mass-vaccination-against-omicron-give-the-final-blow

"To all those who believe Omicron is signaling the transition of the pandemic into endemicity."

Read here:
www.voiceforscienceandsolidarity.org/scientific-blog/to-all-those-who-believe-omicron-is-signaling-the-transition-of-the-pandemic-into-endemicity

"Omicron: A Wolf In Sheep's Clothing."

Read here:
www.voiceforscienceandsolidarity.org/scientific-blog/omicron-a-wolf-in-sheeps-clothing

Charts & Figures

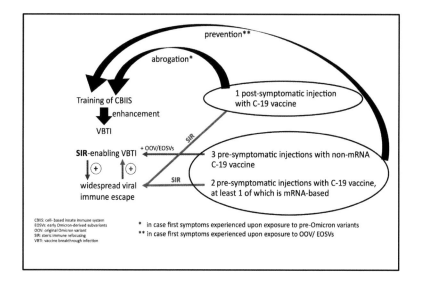

Fig. 1: The impact of C-19 vaccination on immune escape and CBIIS training.

If first C-19 symptoms were experienced upon exposure to pre-Omicron lineages, 1 post-symptomatic injection with an mRNA-based C-19 vaccine was likely sufficient to abrogate training of the CBIIS and to trigger widespread viral immune escape via SIR. If first C-19 symptoms were experienced upon exposure to OOV or EOSVs, 3 pre-symptomatic injections with a non-mRNA-based C-19 vaccine or 2 pre-symptomatic injections with a C-19 vaccine injection, at least one of which is mRNA-based, were likely required to prevent training of the CBIIS and trigger widespread viral immune escape via SIR.

The threshold for triggering SIR is much lower in the case of mRNA-based vaccines. In previously infection-inexperienced individuals, for example, a primary series of C-19 vaccinations comprising a single mRNA-based injection suffices to prevent cell-based innate immune training by triggering SIR directly, regardless of whether administered during the pre-Omicron or Omicron (OOV/ EOSV) stage of the immune escape pandemic.

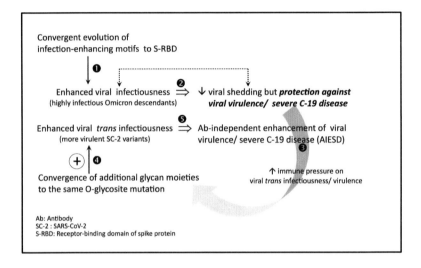

Fig. 2: Exposure to highly infectious Omicron descendants results in diminished viral shedding and a gradual increase in PNNAb-mediated immune pressure on viral virulence.This will likely drive the emergence of new, highly infectious SC-2 variants that are characterized by more extensive/ abundant glycosylation of the O-glycosite mutation and thereby confer a higher level of intrinsic *trans* infectiousness/ virulence.

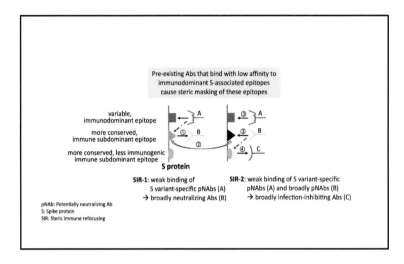

Fig.3: SIR-enabling VBTIs drive large-scale viral immune escape in vaccinees by reorienting the immune response to S-associated antigenic sites that prime broadly functional antibodies (Abs) with low affinity. SIR occurs when pre-existing Abs (A) bind with low affinity to their target epitopes on progeny virus or *in vivo* synthesized vaccinal antigen (i.e., in the case of mRNA transfection), respectively. SIR-induced Abs to subdominant S-associated antigenic domains have low affinity and therefore place high immune pressure on these more conserved domains. SIR therefore allows for fast and large-scale immune escape. SIR-1 triggers induction of broadly neutralizing Abs of low affinity (B) that are directed at more conserved, immune subdominant epitopes (①). This drives large-scale immune escape of SC-2 variants (EOSVs) that are no longer neutralizable (②) and provoke new PNNAb-mediated VBTIs; the latter allow pre-existing pNAbs to bind with low affinity to the S-associated immunodominant or mutated subdominant epitopes expressed on the new progeny virus (A and B, respectively; ③). This triggers SIR-2, which allows other, less immunogenic subdominant S-associated epitopes to prime broadly infection-inhibiting Abs of low affinity (C; ④). The latter drive large-scale emergence of highly infectious Omicron descendants that trigger PNNAb-*independent* VBTIs.

GEERT VANDEN BOSSCHE, DVM, PHD

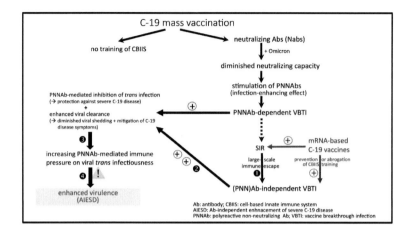

Fig. 4: PNNAb-mediated enhancement of viral infectiousness triggers PNNAb-dependent BTI in C-19 vaccinees and may thereby trigger SIR. SIR-enabling VBTIs promote large-scale immune escape in highly C-19 vaccinated populations and eventually drive widespread (PNN)Ab-independent VBTIs (due to co-circulating highly infectious Omicron descendants) [❶]. Widespread (PNN)Ab-independent VBTIs provide C-19 vaccinees with sustained protection against (severe) C-19 disease and strongly diminishes viral shedding (❷) while gradually causing the highly C-19 vaccinated population to raise PNNAb-mediated immune pressure on viral *trans* infectiousness (❸). This puts C-19 vaccinees at high risk of contracting AIESD (❹).

SIR-enabling mRNA-based C-19 vaccines expedite large-scale viral immune escape while preventing or abrogating training of the CBIIS. It is therefore likely that mRNA vaccination will dramatically enhance the rate of (PNN)Ab-independent VBTIs in highly C-19 vaccinated populations. By causing highly C-19 vaccinated populations to rapidly increase PNNAb-mediated immune pressure after a prolonged lag time, this evolution could eventually lead to the sudden emergence of an extremely virulent SC-2 variant. This suggests that mRNA-vaccinated individuals in highly vaccinated populations are at high risk of contracting AIESD.

⊕ indicates a stimulatory effect

180

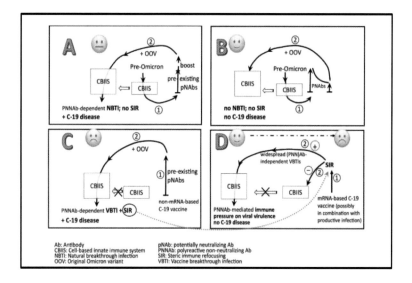

Fig. 5: Trained CBII in the unvaccinated (panels A and B) but not in the C-19 vaccinated (panels C and D) prevents BTIs from triggering SIR.

Panel A: Exposure to OOV shortly after NBTI with a pre-Omicron variant promotes PNNAb-dependent NBTI but does not enable SIR thanks to dampening of the reproduction rate of viral progeny by trained CBII;

Panel B: Alternatively, when exposure to OOV does not occur shortly after previous productive infection with pre-Omicron variants, pNAb concentrations will have declined down to a level that is too low to trigger stimulation of PNNAbs and provoke PNNAb-dependent NBTI.

Panel C: non-mRNA-based C-19 vaccines usually generate higher and prolonged pNAb titers; since C-19 vaccines do not train the CBIIS (since they do not contain replicating virus), C-19 vaccinees are more likely to contract SIR-enabling, PNNAb-dependent VBTIs upon exposure to OOV.

Panel D: mRNA-based C-19 vaccines, alone or in combination with productive infection, trigger SIR on their own (①). They therefore promote sidelining of the CBIIS and eventually expedite widespread

(PNN)Ab-independent VBTIs (②). The latter led to a rise in population-level PNNAb-mediated immune pressure on viral virulence. mRNA-vaccinated individuals in highly mRNA-vaccinated populations are therefore at higher risk of developing AIESD, regardless of whether they had an opportunity to train their CBIIS during the pre-Omicron phase of the immune escape pandemic.

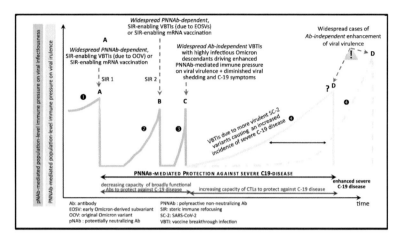

Fig. 6: Reverse molecular epidemiology applied to highly C-19 vaccinated populations. Data from deep mutational scanning (DMS) and immunological characterization of relevant sera can provide information on the evolutionary dynamics of population-level immune pressure placed on viral infectiousness and viral virulence. While the DMS data themselves have little predictive value, monitoring the evolution of population-level immune pressure derived from this data enables the prediction of critical inflection points (A, B, C, D). Whereas PNNAb-dependent VBTIs abruptly diminish humoral immune pressure on variant-specific and variant-nonspecific viral neutralizability (A and B, respectively), PNNAb-independent VBTIs abruptly abolish humoral immune pressure on variant-nonspecific viral infectiousness (C) while causing highly C-19 vaccinated populations to gradually augment humoral immune pressure on viral *trans* infectiousness (❹).

Highly virulent SC-2 variants with highly glycosylated O-glycosite mutations will ultimately abolish this immune pressure (D). ❶❷❸❹ respectively indicate growing pNAb-mediated immune pressure on variant-specific viral infectiousness, variant-nonspecific neutralizability and infectiousness and (variant-nonspecific) virulence.
It is important to note that – as a general rule – the higher the C-19 vaccine coverage rate and the more booster doses are administered, the slower the immune pressure on the virus will grow but the

higher the level of population-immune pressure that will be reached when the concentration and/ or affinity of the responsible Abs collectively decline (after a prolonged lag time). This is thought to particularly apply to highly C-19 vaccinated populations that have been immunized with mRNA-based C-19 vaccines. It is therefore reasonable to predict that these populations will be more likely to experience a substantial wave of AIESD (see dashed yellow line).

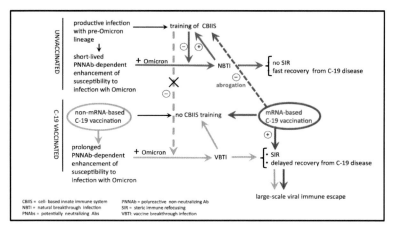

Fig. 7: Productive infection with pre-Omicron lineages results in training of the CBIIS and a short-lived increase in pNAb titers. This prevents subsequent NBTIs with Omicron from enabling SIR and allows them to enhance training of the CBIIS. This is in sharp contrast to C-19 vaccination with non-mRNA-based C-19 vaccines. As those fail to train the CBIIS and induce high pNAb titers, they enable VBTIs with Omicron to cause SIR and thereby enable large-scale immune escape. Once a booster dose has been administered productive infection can no longer prevent Omicron-induced VBTIs from enabling SIR (see dashed green line).

mRNA-based C-19 vaccines trigger SIR and thereby expedite viral immune escape while preventing or abrogating training of the CBIIS upon viral exposure.

⊖ indicates an inhibitory effect whereas ⊕ indicates a stimulatory effect

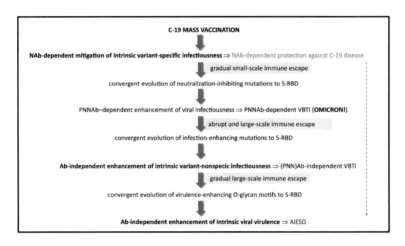

Fig. 8: Flow chart depicting the evolutionary dynamics of SC-2 immune escape as initially triggered by C-19 mass vaccination. The advent of Omicron marked a turning point as SIR-enabling PNNAb-dependent VBTIs mediated transition from NAb-dependent vaccine-mediated <u>mitigation of intrinsic viral infectiousness</u> to Ab-independent <u>enhancement of intrinsic viral infectiousness</u> and thereby fueled Ab-independent VBTIs. The latter facilitate transition from Ab-independent enhancement of intrinsic viral infectiousness to Ab-independent enhancement of intrinsic viral virulence (causing Ab-independent enhancement of severe C-19 disease; AIESD). Because SIR drives viral immune escape, mRNA vaccines expedited the occurrence of PNNAb-dependent VBTIs. It is therefore reasonable to assume that mRNA vaccines will substantially contribute to raising PNNAb-mediated population-level immune pressure on viral virulence in highly mRNA-vaccinated populations. As S-RBD is largely responsible for viral infectiousness and enabling conformational transition that facilitates *trans* fusion (i.e., viral virulence), enhanced intrinsic viral infectiousness and virulence involve convergent evolution of S-RBD. Enhanced intrinsic viral infectiousness involves convergent evolution of amino acid mutations to S-RBD whereas enhanced intrinsic viral virulence will likely involve convergent evolution of glycosidic moieties to O-glycosite mutations comprised within S-RBD (**❺**).

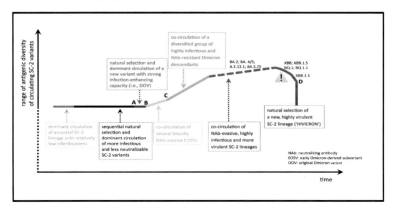

Fig. 9: Population-level immune pressure on more conserved, immunodominant S-associated epitopes promotes fast and large-scale immune escape. A short-lived surge in population-level immune pressure on more conserved, S-associated domains triggers abrupt sequential co-circulation of several antigenically distinct, largely NAb-evasive EOSVs and highly infectious Omicron descendants. Growing population-level immune pressure on viral *trans* infectiousness likely triggers the emergence of a diversified set of highly infectious, NAb-evasive Omicron descendants which gradually expand their O-linked glycosylation to enable a higher level of intrinsic viral virulence.

As enhanced O-glycosylation may cause steric hindrance of viral entry, antigenic diversity of viral variants may suddenly diminish at the advantage of a single immune escape variant that has succeeded in enhancing its virulence without compromising a its enhanced intrinsic infectiousness (e.g., XBB.1.5.). When the overall immune response in highly C-19 vaccinated populations will evolve to cause a sudden surge in population-level immune pressure on viral virulence, a new and unique, highly virulent SC-2 variant will be selected (HIVICRON). The latter will rapidly abrogate the population-level immune pressure by provoking a large wave of AIESD. The inflection points (A, B, C, D) correspond to those depicted in fig. 6.

The names of some relevant, more infectious and more virulent co-circulating (sub)variants are indicated along the red part of the curve.

187

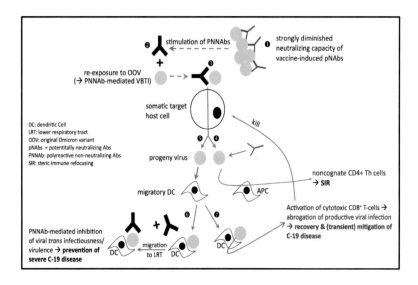

Fig. 10: Pathogenesis of PNNAb-dependent VBTI. Diminished neutralizing capacity of pNAbs to OOV triggers stimulation of PNNAbs (❶❷); binding of PNNAbs to OOV provokes PNNAb-dependent VBTI (❸). pNAbs bind in relatively low concentration to progeny virus because of the enhanced viral production rate in target host cells (❹). As this likely delays uptake of progeny virions into APCs, PNNAb-dependent VBTIs are thought to trigger SIR. PNNAb-mediated enhancement of viral infectiousness further promotes adsorption of infectious progeny virus onto migratory DCs (❺❻), thereby enabling PNNAbs to prevent severe C-19 disease. Abundant uptake of non-adsorbed virus in patrolling DCs/ APCs (❼) ultimately triggers cytotoxic killing of virus-infected host cells and promotes recovery and mitigation of C-19 disease.

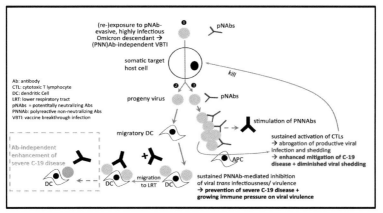

Fig. 11: Pathogenesis of (PNN)Ab-independent VBTI. High intrinsic infectiousness of co-circulating Omicron descendants precipitates infection of target host cells (❶) and enhances the production rate of highly infectious progeny virus. The latter predominantly adsorbs onto tissue-resident DCs and thereby causes pre-existing PNNAbs to only bind in relatively low concentration to progeny virus tethered to migratory DCs (❷). Diminished virulence-inhibiting capacity of pre-existing PNNAbs causes highly C-vaccinated populations to raise immune pressure on viral virulence while still protecting C-19 vaccinees from severe C-19 disease. As enhanced virus adsorption to DCs results in relatively low concentrations of free/ non-adsorbed progeny virions, vaccinal pNAbs bind to the latter in relatively high concentration and thereby trigger stimulation of PNNAbs (❸); Enhanced uptake of multimeric pNAb-virus complexes into patrolling APCs strongly activates cytotoxic T cells (CTLs) enabling killing of virus-infected host cells. Large-scale Ab-independent VBTIs likely promote prolonged mitigation of C-19 disease symptoms and reduced viral shedding. As vaccinal pNAb titers decline slowly (especially after booster shots), production of PNNAbs will be re-stimulated upon re-exposure of C-19 vaccinees to (large-scale) Ab-independent VBTIs; this will slow down the growth of PNNAb-mediated population-level immune pressure on viral virulence. However, widespread decline of pNAb titers will ultimately cause the highly C-19 vaccinated population to abruptly increase its immune pressure on viral virulence. This is thought to trigger selection of a new, highly virulent SC-2 variant that enables large-scale occurrence of Ab-independent enhancement of severe C-19 disease (AIESD).

189

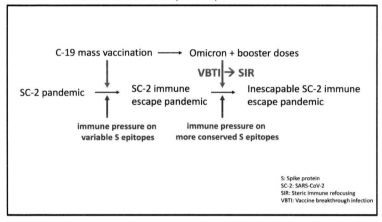

Fig. 12: How C-19 mass vaccination during the SC-2 pandemic turned a natural pandemic into an inescapable SC-2 immune escape pandemic.

Addendum

[1] Insufficient cell-based innate immune capacity can also be due to a poor health status (e.g., in the case of co-morbidities)

[2] In my opinion, cases of classical Ab-dependent enhancement of C-19 disease exclusively occurred during the pre-Omicron phase of the SC-2 immune escape pandemic. This is because ADE is triggered by exposure of high titers of pre-existing high-affinity Abs to an antigenically drifted viral variant. However, binding of pre-existing Abs with low affinity to a heterologous viral variant (e.g., decorated with an antigenically 'shifted' S protein) or binding of low-affinity Abs to a homologous viral variant is thought to precipitate productive infection of target host cells while sparing APCs and thereby preserving the professional capacity of these cells to present antigen.

[3] Provision of T help enables Bc antigens to prime immunological memory whereas Th-independent antigens do not prime memory B cells. Th-independent antigens/ epitopes are therefore weakly immunogenic and the Abs they elicit are short-lived.

[4] 'immunocryptic' epitopes relate to antigenic motifs that are hidden and not usually immunogenic unless the protein they are part of engages in conformational changes that make them recognizable by the host immune system. Multimeric clustering of the Ag carrier may, for example, enable presentation of surface-expressed immunocryptic epitopes in a repetitive array and thereby render them immunogenic.

[5] One can only speculate about the Th-independent nature of S antigen expressed at the surface of SC-2-infected or mRNA-transfected cells. It is likely however that prior to its incorporation into viral particles or release from mRNA-transfected cells, cell surface-expressed trimeric S protein presents in repetitive patterns at the surface of these cells.

[6] During natural infection, viral protein expressed at the surface of virus-infected cells cannot prime an immune response because the virus (but not mRNA-based vaccine constructs!) synthesizes peptides that prevent antigen presentation by cognate APCs at an early stage of infection. Hence, no cognate CD4+ T helper cells are induced. In the absence of effective assistance by T helper cells, S

protein that is transiently expressed on the surface of SC-2-infected cells cannot prime an immune response.

[7] *Trans* infection has been reported to strongly correlate with viral *trans* fusion and the occurrence of syncytia. The latter are pathognomonic for severe C-19 disease

[8] I have previously predicted that these mutations would involve an altered glycosylation profile of S protein (ref. 5)

[9] Except in those who only became exposed to the new emerging, highly infectious Omicron descendants at a time where their short-lived PNNAbs had already reached suboptimal virulence-inhibitory levels, C-19 disease symptoms in vaccinated individuals are now substantially mitigated upon re-exposure to all circulating SC-2 variants

[10] Although broadly cross-functional memory B cells eventually acquire memory, it takes several months of affinity-maturation in germinal centers before they achieve full-fledged memory and affinity

[11] However, BTIs also occurred in unvaccinated individuals who became exposed to OOV or EOSVs shortly after previous productive infection with a pre-Omicron variant. These individuals were prone to developing PNNAb-dependent NBTI because their naturally induced, S variant-specific Abs were a poor match OOV or EOSVs.

[12] The statements and insights shared in this chapter are largely based on my interpretation and analysis of data reported in numerous publications, a non-exhaustive list of which is published at the end of this book (refs. 13-32)

[13] Antigenic motifs that present in polymeric arrays are known to be able to restimulate previously primed memory B cells and recall affinity-matured Abs towards Th-independent epitopes (this is how subjects primed with polysaccharide conjugate vaccines recall full-fledged Abs upon subsequent encounter with *Streptococcus* bacteria coated with Th-independent polysaccharides)

[14] Cell surface-expressed S protein may trigger complement activation and inflammatory cytokine cascades in tissue cells expressing S protein at their surface and thereby provoke organ-specific inflammation-associated disease => staat op pagina 42

[15] https://www.ncbi.nlm.nih.gov/pmc/articles/PMC4868770/

[16] mRNA-based C-19 vaccination after infection-mediated or C-19 vaccine-mediated priming of CD4+ T helper cells is likely to prime low-affinity memory B cells and trigger SIR upon subsequent viral exposure

[17] adapted mRNA bivalent vaccines target the ancestral Wujhan-Hu strain and newly emerged Omicron-derived subvariants (e.g., BA.4-5 subvariants)

[18] OOV incorporated over 30 single point mutations, 15 of which occurred in the S-RBD (ref. 6)

[19] In analogy with low-affinity variant S-specific Abs, it is reasonable to assume that anti-S Abs that bind with low affinity to more conserved domains within S-NTD exhibit broadly (i.e., variant-nonspecific) 'infection-inhibiting' activity

[20] These mutations consist of specific epitopes that were responsible for enhanced intrinsic infectiousness of specific pre-Omicron SC-2 variants (e.g., Beta, Gamma, and Delta lineages).

[21] Large-scale population-level immune pressure may have led to natural selection of a distinct subset of Omicron-derived [sub]variants in distinct highly C-19 vaccinated populations. This contributes to the overall diversity of currently co-circulating SC-2 variants across highly C-19 vaccinated countries/ regions. Highly infectious Omicron [sub]variants selected in one given highly C-19 vaccinated population could mix with those selected in another highly vaccinated population.

[22] As previously reported, this conserved antigenic site is responsible for trans infection of SC-2 virions tethered to migratory DCs (5)

[23] Antigenic determinants mediating enhanced intrinsic infectiousness of previously circulating pre-Omicron variants (e.g., Beta, Gamma and Delta variant)

[24] This is because affinity maturation of the recalled Abs is delayed by several months (relative to the time point of the VBTI or mRNA booster dose)

[25] By occurring in 2 different stages, competition between broadly functional Abs of different affinity can be avoided. As protection against productive infection following repeated Omicron-induced VBTIs or mRNA-based booster injections rapidly vanished, it is, indeed, reasonable to assume that SIR 2-mediated priming yielded Abs of lower affinity (than those induced by SIR 1) against S-NTD domains that are even more conserved than those previously recognized by SIR 1-induced Abs

[26] The statements and insights shared in this subchapter are largely based on my interpretation and analysis of data reported in numerous publications, a non-exhaustive list of which is published at the end of this book. (13-32)

[27] Because of their Th independence, PNNAbs do not undergo affinity-maturation.

[28] PNNAbs prevent infectious SC-2 virions adsorbed onto migratory DCs from being transferred to SC-2-permissive host cells in distal organs

[29] for as long as viral uptake into APCs does not suffice to sustain activation of MHC class I-unrestricted CTLs, C-19 vaccinated individuals would only be protected against severe C-19 disease (via PNNAbs; fig. 10).

[30] This implies that killing would also affect unvaccinated individuals, even those whose CBIIS is adequately trained

[31] Diminished transmission is due to reduced viral shedding and infectiousness of recently emerged Omicron descendants (57)

[32] The larger the population and the higher the relative contribution of immunologically naïve individuals (i.e., not previously exposed people such as young children), the higher the likelihood that SC-2 can spread through asymptomatic transmission despite established herd immunity

[33] In a previous contribution, I explained how O-glycosite mutations on S protein would allow the virus to enhance its virulence. It is plausible, but unproven, that more abundantly glycosylated O-glycosite mutations will enable a high level of intrinsic viral virulence. Alike with OOV, a spectacular shift is expected to occur suddenly when population-level immune pressure mounts beyond a certain threshold. This is likely to occur

when a unique S-associated O-glycosite mutation will eventually be selected when PNNAb titers in a highly C-19 vaccinated population evolve to exert high population-level immune pressure on viral virulence.

[34] It goes without saying that loss of protection against viral virulence will automatically cause loss of protection against C-19 disease altogether. This is because unlocked viral virulence of highly infectious variants will cause a massive enhancement of viral *trans* infectiousness resulting in viral dissemination to distal organs (i.e., due to Ab-independent enhancement of severe C-19 disease).

[35] I expect the first waves of highly virulent virus to manifest in regions that rapidly proceeded with mass vaccination (i.e., beginning of 2021) but had only limited booster doses (e.g., UK) and/ or primarily used mRNA-based C-19 vaccines (e.g., Israel, USA, several European countries). As the latter trigger SIR by themselves, it is reasonable to expect that massive deployment of these vaccines will have limited the window of opportunity for vaccinated individuals to train their CBIIS while having expedited viral immune escape dynamics. Populations vaccinated with mRNA-based C-19 vaccines are therefore likely to not only be the first (to be) affected by more virulent SC-2 variants but to also record the highest C-19 hospitalization and mortality rates.

[36] Booster shots will initially boost vaccine-induced pNAbs or cross-neutralizing Abs (the latter in the case of SIR) and thereby ensure re-stimulation of PNNAbs upon re-exposure

[37] Omicron descendants are not only spreading in the human population but also in animal reservoirs and even in bacterial cells (ref. 54)

[38] These C-19 surges of severe disease are, however, likely to coincide with surges in other acute self-limiting diseases as I previously predicted (ref. 5)

[39] PNNAb-mediated BTIs following exposure to highly infectious Omicron variants shortly after recovery from a productive EOSV infection caused more respiratory disease in the unvaccinated, presumably due to a higher level of intrinsic viral infectiousness

[40] Because of their low-affinity, pNAbs in breakthrough-infection convalescents rapidly lost their neutralizing activity against new subvariants (e.g., BA.4.6, BA.2.75.2)

[41] Highly infectious viruses will strongly adsorb on migratory DCs. The minority of free, non-adsorbed progeny virions will therefore bind a relatively higher concentration of pre-existing pNAbs and hence, favor production of virulence-inhibiting PNNAbs while enhancing viral clearance (via CTLs)

[42] In a previous contribution (5), I had called this new variant 'NEWCO'. However, since it still largely inherits its NAb-evasiveness from OOV, the name HIVICRON may be more appropriate

[43] Although antigenically distinct HIVICRON lineages may emerge in different world regions, they will share the same virulence-enhancing mutation

[44] In case of highly infectious Omicron descendants, binding of pNAbs to these new variants will <u>no longer occur before</u> (PNNAb-dependent) VBTI <u>but after</u> (Ab-independent) VBTI.

[45] Given diminished viral transmissibility, exposure of the vast majority of unvaccinated individuals to highly infectious variants further contributed to training of their CBIIS and elicited at most some mild C-19 disease symptoms

[46] This particularly applies to the mRNA-based vaccines

[47] Because pNAbs protected against disease from new variants without protecting against infection, mass C-19 vaccination drove dominant propagation of new, more infectious pre-Omicron variants

[48] Even though C-19 vaccination shortly after natural infection is not recommended, vaccination with any mRNA-based C-19 vaccine at any time after symptomatic or even asymptomatic/ mild infection likely promotes SIR; post-infection vaccination with an mRNA-based C-19 vaccine is therefore always supposed/ expected to discontinue innate immune training of NK cells upon exposure to new emerging SC-2 variants

[49] In this case, 'vaccinated' refers to a person who received 2 or more doses of a C-19 vaccine

[50] This could also apply to C-19 vaccinated individuals who managed to preserve training capacity in the course of this pandemic. This primarily applies to those who received no more than 2 doses of a non-mRNA-based C-19 vaccine prior to developing C-19 disease

[51] Bivalent vaccines are targeting both the ancestral strain as well as Omicron-derived variants such as the Omicron BA.4/BA.5 variant
[52] In the current stage of the pandemic (highly infectious, co-circulating variants), the administration of Omicron-adapted booster doses would even be totally obsolete as Ab-independent VBTIs do not allow for priming of new Abs (see chapter...).
[53] Short-lived protection against productive infection led to short-term reduction of viral transmission and delayed viral immune escape. This explains why I have underestimated the timeline for more virulent variants to emerge

[54] Diminished protection or enhanced susceptibility in the unvaccinated was certainly also partially due to the infection-enhancing activity of short-lived (6-8 weeks), non-neutralizing IgM Abs in previously asymptomatically infected individuals. This is because enhanced viral infection rates increase the likelihood for an unvaccinated person to become rapidly re-exposed after previous asymptomatic infection, i.e., at a point in time where the infection-enhancing IgM is still quite high.
[55] i.e., vaccination after previous productive infection with a pre-Omicron variant or after previous C-19 vaccination, or a booster dose after a primary series of mRNA vaccination
[56] In the case of Omicron, enhanced infectiousness was mediated by PNNAb Abs
[57] In the absence of re-infection, adsorbed particles will presumably end up being internalized into APCs and therefore continue to outcompete other Ags. At a population level this may suffice to prolong the effect of re-exposure. This postulate seems to be confirmed by the observation that vaccines experience continued protection from C-19 disease despite the short-lived activity of activated MHC class I-unrestricted CTLs. Given the high level of viral

infectiousness and lack of symptoms (asymptomatic transmission!),
it seems unlikely that *de novo* priming with a new Ag (requiring at
least 2 interspaced injections) would not be interrupted by re-
exposure

[58] due to PNNAb-mediated inhibition of viral *trans* infectiousness/
virulence

[59] due to *de novo* induction of cross-functional Abs following SIR-
enabling VBTI or administration of an mRNA-based vaccine booster
dose.

[60] As these mutations replaced the conserved targeted regions, they
were no longer a good match to the broadly functional Abs that had
been elicited as a result of SIR-enabling VBTIs triggered by OOV/
EOSVs.

[61] It is important to understand that during the pre-Omicron phase,
individuals who developed asymptomatic/ mild symptoms
following SC-2 exposure could develop more serious C-19
symptoms upon viral re-exposure shortly (i.e., within 6-8 weeks)
after their primary infection. This is thought to be due to the
infection-enhancing effect of short-lived, non-neutralizing IgM Abs.
The more infectious the dominantly circulating virus, the higher the
likelihood of re-exposure shortly after the primary infection.
Likewise, re-exposure to an antigenically *shifted* variant within a few
months after previous infection with a more distant SC-2 variant
could trigger PNNAb-dependent BTI in unvaccinated individuals
because of insufficient neutralizing Ab capacity. In both cases,
unvaccinated people contracted C-19 disease despite a trained
CBIIS. In both cases, C-19 disease in the unvaccinated was due to
rapid re-infection by dominantly circulating, more infectious SC-2
variants that were selected because of population-level immune
pressure on S protein (i.e., on viral infectiousness). As these
phenomena typically occurred in highly C-19 vaccinated
populations, there is no doubt that mass vaccination with S protein-
based C-19 vaccines has been responsible for relapse of C-19 disease
in unvaccinated individuals who previously experienced productive
SC-2 infection.

[62] Widespread suboptimal immune pressure on viral infectiousness
and neutralizability typically results from mass vaccination during a

pandemic, using vaccines that are directed at the protein that is responsible for viral infection and neutralization (i.e., S protein in the case of SC-2)

[63] Masking relates to the binding of Ag to cognate Abs that do no longer bind strongly enough to the Ag to outcompete ACE2 for binding to the viral S-RBD but still bind with sufficient strength to prevent the Ag from being recognized by previously primed B memory cells

[64] More immunogenic (immunodominant) domains that co-localize with less immunogenic antigenic sites will outcompete the latter for assistance from cognate memory T helper cells

[65] It is important to note that NAbs primed by natural infection do not last for as long as C-19 vaccine-induced NAbs. PNNAb-dependent NBTIs could therefore only occur within a relatively short time window (4-6w) after previous infection.

[66] This is because most of the highly infectious progeny virus likely binds to migratory DCs (ref. 40)

[67] Changes to the 'conserved' antigenic site would threaten viral reproduction because this antigenic site is critically important for the virus to enable enhancement of its infectiousness and trigger PNNAb-mediated BTIs (regardless of the variant) in case its survival is threatened by population-level immunity.

[68] As explained in chapter 4.3. this situation has recently changed due to enhanced virulence of circulating Omicron descendants

[69] This also implies that there is no reason for the unvaccinated to avoid contact with C-19 vaccinated individuals.

[70] As discussed under 11.9, enhanced prevalence of other diseases in C-19 vaccines is thought to be due to enhanced SC-2 uptake into APCs. Enhanced virus uptake into APCs may cause diminished presentation of other pathogen-derived Ags by these APCs and therefore prevent recall or priming of effector B and T cells that depend on CD4+ T help.

About Geert Vanden Bossche, DVM, PHD

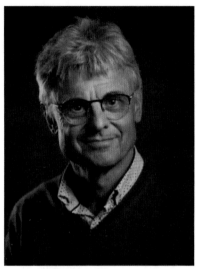

portrait by Berten.be

Dr. Vanden Bossche received his DVM from the University of Ghent, Belgium, and his PHD degree in Virology from the University of Hohenheim, Germany. He held adjunct faculty appointments at universities in Belgium and Germany. After his career in Academia, Geert joined several vaccine companies (GSK Biologicals, Novartis Vaccines, Solvay Biologicals) to serve various roles in vaccine R&D as well as in late vaccine development. Geert then moved on to join the Bill & Melinda Gates Foundation's Global Health Discovery team in Seattle (USA) as Senior Program Officer. He then worked with the Global Alliance for Vaccines and Immunization (GAVI) in Geneva as Senior Ebola Program Manager and subsequently joined the German Center for Infection Research in Cologne as Head of the Vaccine Development Office.

Geert is now primarily serving as a Biotech/Vaccine consultant while also conducting his own research on Natural Killer cell-based vaccines.

As a creative thinker, innovator, entrepreneur and visionary, Geert has been invited to speak at multiple international congresses. His work and supportive advice are driven by a relentless passion to translate scientific breakthrough findings into competitive solutions to emerging challenges in public and global health. Dr. Vanden Bossche has become world famous for warning Humanity against the health danger of conducting mass vaccination programs during a pandemic (March 2021).

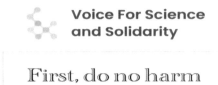

Voice For Science and Solidarity

Our mission is to unveil and widely share the scientific truths concerning the detrimental health and social consequences of a COVID-19 mass vaccination program conducted during a pandemic.

Proponents of these campaigns largely underestimate the negative impact of widespread immune pressure on both the evolutionary capacity of the virus and the innate immune response.

Worldwide governments' concerted efforts to administer vaccines on a global scale will only prolong the pandemic and lead to catastrophic consequences. Their methods of misinformation and coercion only deepen the magnitude of such a catastrophe and have been accompanied by an increasing erosion of individual rights and freedoms.

Only through global awareness and science-based understanding of these truths through transparency and open scientific debate can we realize the absurdity of this global experiment and pursue a better way forward for humanity.

Geert Vanden Bossche

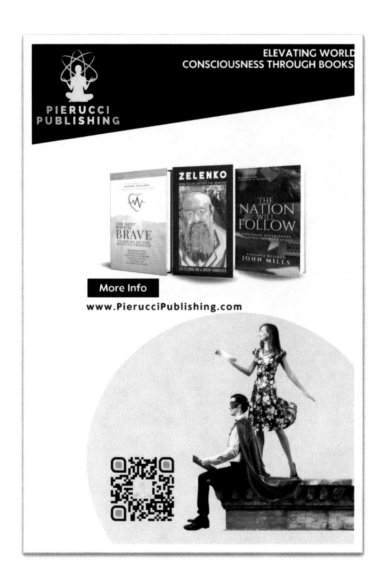